LIVE LONGER LOVE LONGER PART 3

Age is a Treatable Disease

G SYED MD

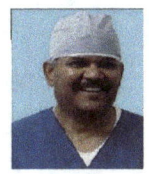

Copyright © 2024 G SYED MD

All rights reserved

The characters and events portrayed in this book are scientific research-based. Any similarity to real persons, living or dead, is coincidental and not intended by the author.

No part of this book may be reproduced, stored in a retrieval system, or transmitted in any form or by any means, electronic, mechanical, photocopying, recording, or otherwise, without express written permission of the publisher.

ISBN: 9798320598109
Imprint: Independently published

Cover design by: Art Painter
Library of Congress Control Number: 2018675309
Printed in the United States of America

Dedicated to the Umar Syed Foundation,

Your mission is so noble, that even Santa Claus asked for a grant application form. Seriously though, your dedication to education and health for indigent communities is like the superhero of nonprofits – saving the day, one stethoscope and textbook at a time.

We're donating the earnings from the Book Series "Live Longer and Love Longer" because, let's face it, laughter is the best medicine, but education and healthcare come pretty close. So here's to helping families and kids suffering from mental illnesses with addiction – may they find the strength to laugh a little louder and love a little longer. Keep doing what you do best – making the world a better place, one belly laugh and prescription refill at a time.

With giggles and gratitude, Love Longevity: Treatable Aging

LIVE LONGER
LOVE LONGER
Part 3
Age is a Treatable Disease

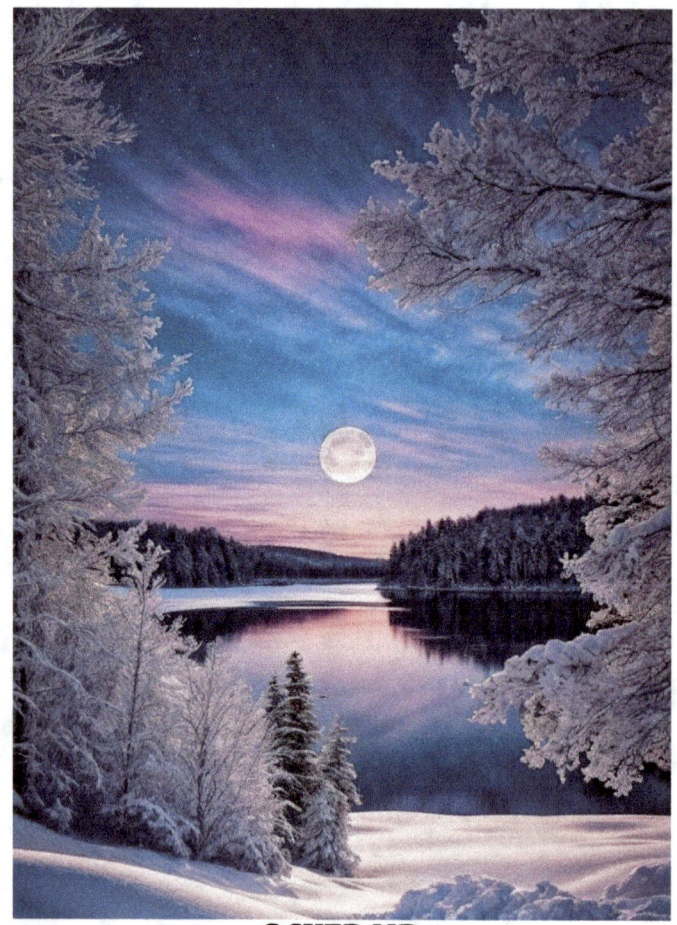

G SYED MD

TABLE OF CONTENT

Preface
Introduction
Chapter 1
- Aging Revolution Ahead
- The Death of Death
- Let's Do Some Numbers
- Wasteful Mother Earth Warning!
- Survival of the Funniest
- Climate Crisis Comedy Hour- Social Injustice
- Riches and wrinkles forever

Chapter 2
- People Overflow, Birth Control
- Epic Quest: Defeat Aging!
- Age Defiance- Future Potential
- Funding for Research

Chapter 3
- Fix Senior's Tooth Trouble
- Cosmic Lifespan and Euthnasia
- GMO train
- Gene Editing
- Tech Eco Adventure Saga
- Generation United: Embrace Futur
- Code MG2A: Old Age
- Daily Health Tips
- The Saga of Supplements
- My Golden Years

Chapter 4

- Aging is a Treatable Disease
- Activate Longevity Genes By
- Personalized Medicine Program
- Gene Technologies
- Hayflick Limit
- NANOG: Master of all Genes
- Chromosomal (Nullbar) Mutations
- Toxic "Senescent Zombies" Cells
- Cell Loss and Atrophy

Chapter 5
- Emerging Technologies Nanotech Revived Cell
- Genetic Risk Profile
- Telemedicine Consult Virtual Medical Advice
- Regenerative Medicine
- http://www.inxstatetracker.com

Chapter 6
- Gene Defects (Genomics)
- Autism: A Genetic Defects
- Single Nucleotide Polymorphism

Chapter 7
- Environmental DNA Damager
- Carcinogens.
- Airport Noise
- Cool CRISPR Cancer Fight!
- Ribosome Switch Technology (Riboswitch)

Chapter 8
- Dementia: Mini-Mental-State Summary
- Title: Fun Brain Quiz Adventure!
- For Brain Power Over 60 Years of Age
- Behavioral Variant Frontotemporal Dementia

Chapter 9
- Breakthrough Technology
- Innovative Technologies
- Aging Technologies Revolution

Riboswitch
Incredible Breakthroughs in Healthcare!
Platelet-Rich Plasma (PRP) Therapy

Chapter 10
Breakthrough Medication: Revolutionary Anti-aging Medication
Stem Cell Therapy
Semaglutide: For Diabetic and Weight Control.

Chapter 11
GOD's Love Anyway
Suffering
Spiritual Weaponry: Combating Deception
The Dynamic Force of Prayer
Fortifying Faith: A Spiritual Arsenal for Life's Challenges
Daily Mindful Meditation for Wellness
The Kingdom of Heaven
Edgar Cayce's Meditation Method
Edgar Cayce's Method of Meditation

Chapter 12
Diet for Higher Consciöusness
Gift For The Day: Happy Life Tips
Personal Hygiene: Hygiene Essential for Senior
Safety/Peace Of Mind
COVID Rules
References and Glossary

Epilogue
Umar Syed RIP 1992-2016

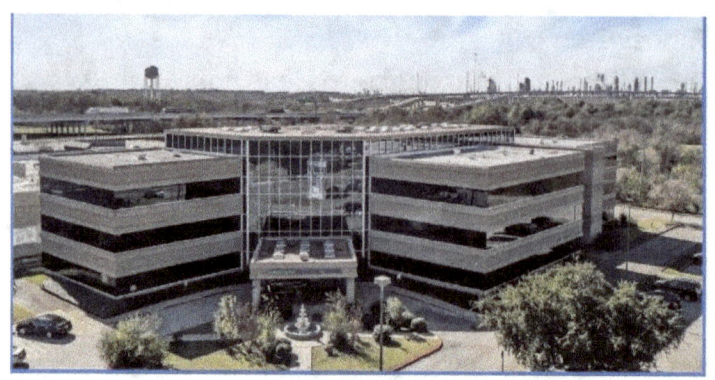

Dedicated to the Umar Syed Foundation,

Your mission is so noble, that even Santa Claus asked for a grant application form. Seriously though, your dedication to education and health for indigent communities is like the superhero of nonprofits – saving the day, one stethoscope and textbook at a time.

We're donating the earnings from the Book Series "Live Longer and Love Longer" because, let's face it, laughter is the best medicine, but education and healthcare come pretty close. So here's to helping families and kids suffering from mental illnesses with addiction – may they find the strength to laugh a little louder and love a little longer. Keep doing what you do best – making the world a better place, one belly laugh and prescription refill at a time.

With giggles and gratitude, Love Longevity: Treatable Aging

LIVE LONGER LOVE LONGER PART 3

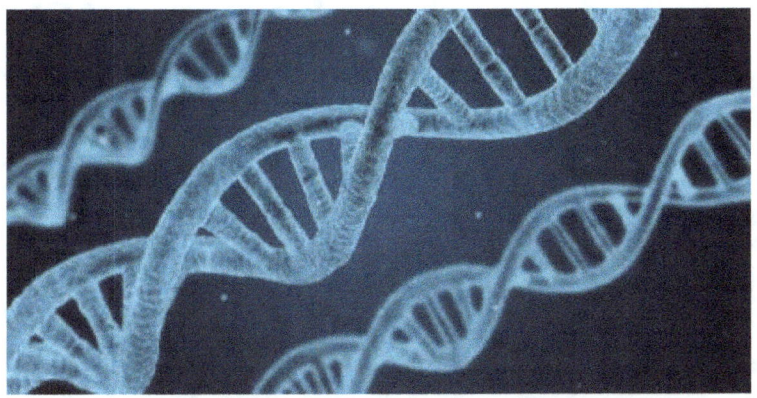

Love Longevity: Treatable Aging
"Extend Your Existence, Extend Your Romance:
Chronicling Aging as a Curable Malady"

Life Expectancy

A statistical measure of the average time a person or group of people are expected to live.

We can use the term for different species of organisms

Human
67 years

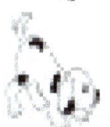
Dog
10-13 years

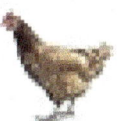
Chicken
8 years

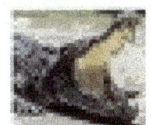
Nile Crocodile
100 years

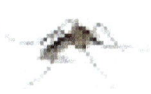
Male Mosquito
10 days

Ranges from 49 years in Swaziland to 83 years in Japan

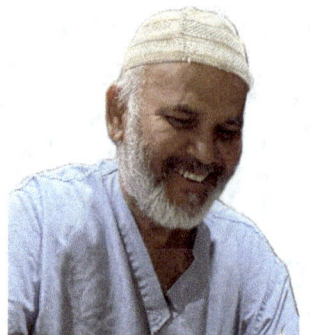

G Syed MD

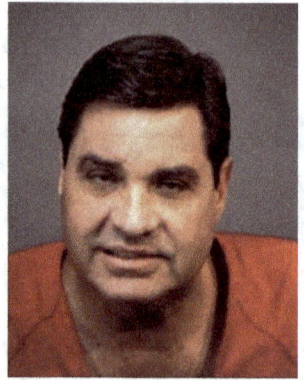

John M. Gayden Jr. MD

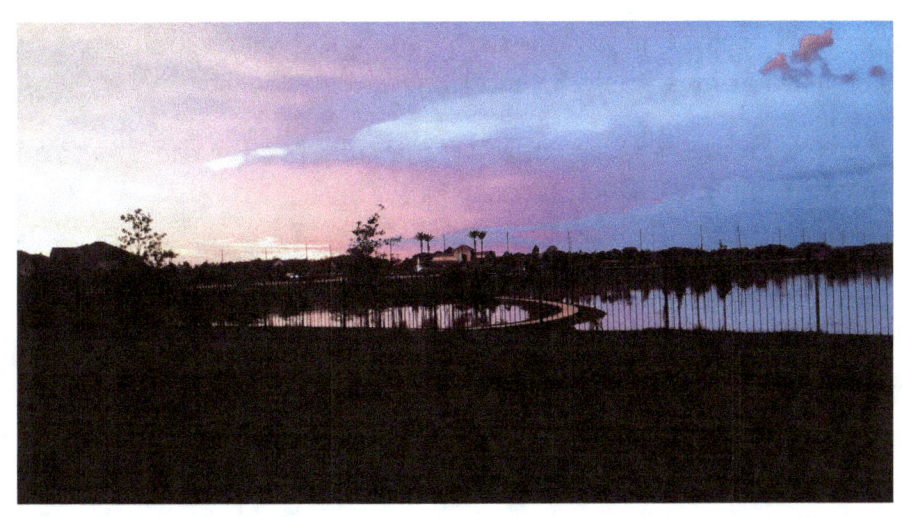

PREFACE

Epic Aging Adventure

Welcome, dear readers, to the uproarious adventure that is "Live Longer, Love Longer, Part 3: Aging is a Treatable Disease"!

If you've ever caught yourself staring in the mirror, contemplating the mysteries of aging, or found yourself muttering, "Why can't I just stay young forever?" then this book is your ticket to the fountain of youth (or at least a good chuckle about it).

In these pages, we're diving headfirst into the wild world of anti-aging science with all the enthusiasm of a kid in a candy store (albeit a kid who's looking for wrinkle cream instead of sweets).

Gone are the days of resigning ourselves to the inevitable march of time – we're flipping the script on aging faster than you can say, "I swear I was just 25 yesterday!"

Prepare yourselves for a rollercoaster ride through the latest and greatest in longevity research.

From stem cells making a Lazarus-like comeback to gene therapies that sound like they're straight out of science fiction (but are totally real, we promise), we're leaving no stone unturned in our quest to unlock the secrets of staying forever young.

But hey, it's not all serious science talk here – we're throwing in a healthy dose of humor to keep things light and breezy. Because let's face it, laughing is probably the best anti-aging remedy out there (that and a good moisturizer).

So, buckle up, folks, and get ready for a journey that's equal parts informative and hilarious. By the time you reach the end of this book, you'll be armed with all the knowledge you need to tackle aging like a boss – and maybe even crack a smile or two along the way.

Now, without further ado, let's dive headfirst into the wacky world of aging and see if we can't wrangle ourselves a few extra years of fun in the sun (or at least a few fewer wrinkles)!

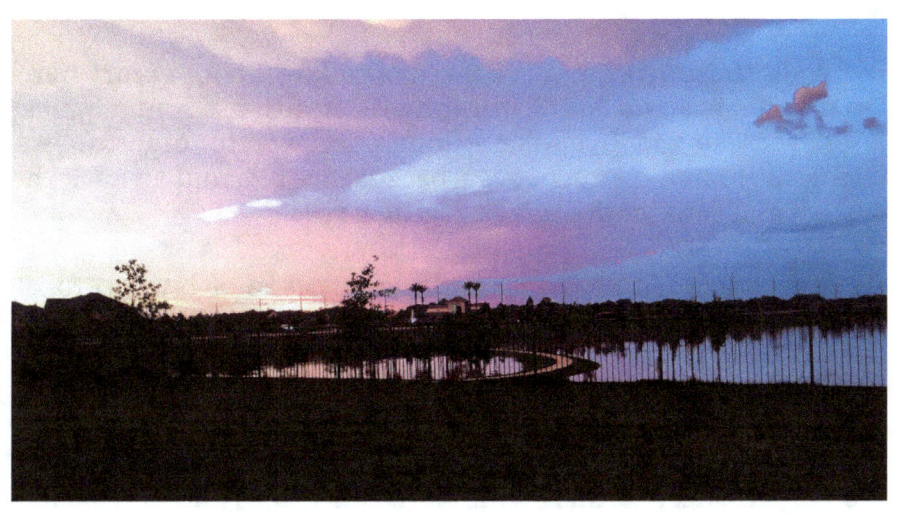

INTRODUCTION

Welcome, fellow time-travelers on the path to perpetual youth and endless laughter!

In the rollicking pages of "Live Longer, Love Longer Part 3: Aging is a Treatable Disease," we're about to embark on a journey so thrilling, it'll make Peter Pan look like he's aged a millennium!

Buckle up, because we're diving headfirst into the fountain of youth, armed with cutting-edge science, a dash of humor, and enough optimism to make Pollyanna blush. Yes, you heard right! We're flipping the script on aging faster than Benjamin Button on a bungee cord.

From the latest anti-aging concoctions that'll have you looking fresher than a daisy at dawn to the wildest predictions about a future where wrinkles are as rare as a unicorn sighting, this book is your ticket to the eternal carnival of youthfulness.

But wait, there's more! We're not just talking about vanity here. Oh no, this is about living our longest, healthiest, and happiest lives ever. Say goodbye to achy joints, farewell to forgetfulness, and adios to age-related woes – because we're about to hack the system and rewrite the rules of aging itself!

So grab your reading glasses and your sense of humor, folks, because we're about to embark on a rollercoaster ride through the wondrous world of regenerative medicine, genetic wizardry, and enough tips for living well to make even Mother Nature jealous.

It's time to defy Father Time and dance into the sunset like there's no tomorrow – because when it comes to aging, the future is looking brighter than a supernova at a disco party.

Get ready to laugh, learn, and live longer than you ever thought possible. Let the adventure begin!

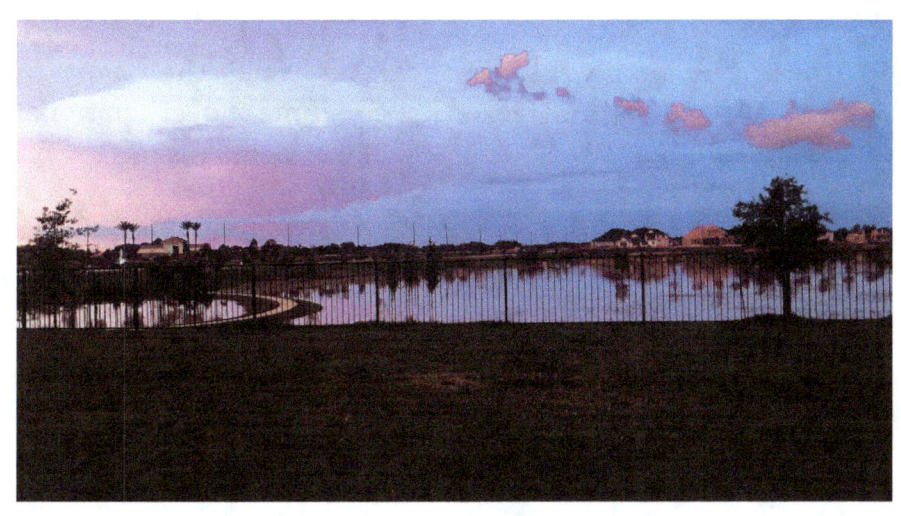

CHAPTER 1

Aging Revolution Ahead

"Immortality for Dummies": A Sneak Peek into the Future, Hilariously Simplified

Alright, picture this: it's 2024, and we're diving into the secrets of living longer, healthier lives.

We're talking about what aging looks like, how to delay it, and even a glimpse into a future where kicking the bucket might be optional!

So, these two brainy genetic engineers spill the beans in Barcelona: by 2045, they reckon we could make death optional and reverse aging.

Yep, you heard it right reverse aging! No more creaky joints or saggy skin. We're talking about a world where we're all rocking our best selves for way longer.

And hey, this isn't just some sci-fi dream. These guys are knee-deep in the science stuff, so they know what they're talking about.

Sure, some folks might be skeptical, but the writing's on the wall – longer, healthier lives are on the horizon.

Now, let's think about what this means for society. It's not just about staying sprayed for longer (though that's pretty cool). It's about the potential to achieve more, work longer, and make the most out of life.

Longevity isn't something to be scared of; it's something to embrace with open arms.

So, buckle up, folks! We're on a wild ride to a future where we're all living our best, longest lives ever.

Get ready for some epic adventures ahead!

LIVE LONGER LOVE LONGER PART 3

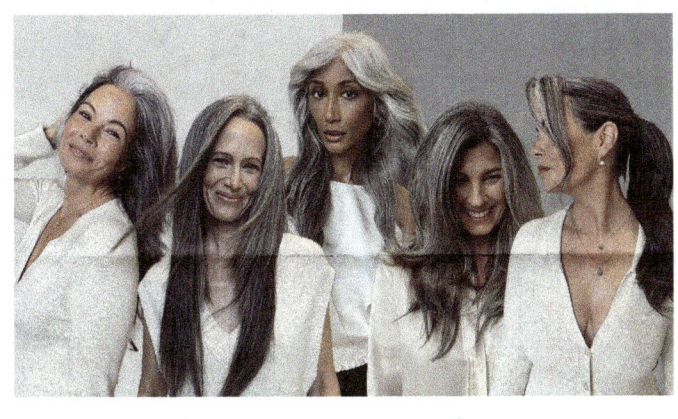

◆ ◆ ◆

The Death of Death

Hold onto your hats, folks! In a twist crazier than a sci-fi flick, genetic masterminds José L. Cordeiro and D. Wood have dropped a bombshell: dying is so last century.

Picture this: they're strutting their stuff in Barcelona, Spain, unveiling their blockbuster book "The Death of Death" like a pair of rockstar scientists.

And what do they bring to the table? Only the most mind-blowing news since sliced bread.

1. Dying Optional, Aging Reversible: Move over, wrinkles! José and David are rewriting the aging rulebook.

They're the Spielberg and Tarantino of genetic engineering, promising a future where aging is about as troublesome as a bad haircut. Benjamin Button, eat your heart out.

2. Old Age as an Illness: Wrinkles? Gray hair?

According to these two, it's all just one big illness waiting to be cured. Taxpayer money for the Fountain of Youth? Count us in!

3. Nanotechnology to the Rescue: Cue the superhero music – nanotech to the rescue!

Dead cells?

Bad genes?

These tiny robots have got your back. It's like having a DIY repair kit for your body.

4. Cordeiro's Anti-Death Pact: José ain't playing by the rules. He's making a bold statement: no death club for him, thank you very much.

In 30 years, he'll be younger. Talk about a life hack!

5. Immortality Doesn't Mean Overcrowding: Don't worry, Earth won't turn into one giant mosh pit.

With space condos on the horizon and fewer rugrats running around, the party can keep on going without the housing crisis.

6. Anti-Aging Treatments vs. Smartphones: Move over, iPhones! José says staying forever young will soon be as trendy as owning the latest gadget.

And hopefully, it'll last longer than your average smartphone.

7. Illegally Immortal in Colombia: They're not just talking the talk; they're walking the walk.

Testing their techniques in Colombia, where regulations are as loose as a magician's morals, these guys are rewriting the rulebook – regulations be damned!

◆ ◆ ◆

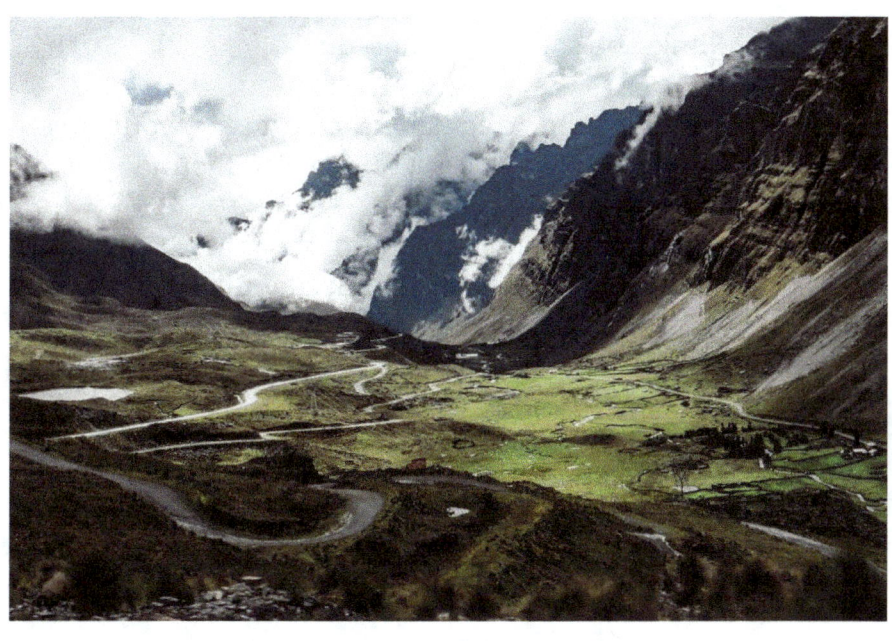

◆ ◆ ◆

Let's Do Some Numbers

L et's embark on a journey of suspenseful speculation, shall we? Buckle up, because we're about to crunch some numbers – but not just any numbers, oh no, these are the kind that might just blow your mind.

Imagine a world where DNA monitoring becomes your very own health whisperer, alerting doctors to diseases before they even think about wreaking havoc.

Cancer? Ha, caught it years before it could even think about making itself known.

Infections? Blink, and they're diagnosed.

Your car seat detects an irregular heartbeat, and your breath analyzer sniffs out immune diseases like a bloodhound.

Even your keyboard is in on the action, tipping off early signs of Parkinson's or multiple sclerosis. Talk about living in a world where your body is constantly under surveillance!

Doctors become like modern-day Sherlock Holmes, armed with more information than they know what to do with – and they get it long before you even set foot in their office.

Medical mishaps? Misdiagnoses? Say goodbye to those nightmares.

But hold onto your hats, because here comes the kicker: let's say all these fancy advancements only give us a measly decade of extra life.

A decade!

But hey, let's not stop there.

What if we all collectively decide that aging isn't our cup of tea and start taking care of ourselves like never before? Suddenly, eating healthier, moving more, and embracing the great outdoors become as trendy as the latest viral TikTok dance. Those lifestyle changes alone could tack on another five years of vitality.

Now, let's sprinkle in some molecules that kick our survival instincts into high gear, giving us a hearty boost of 10 percent more healthy years. That's eight more years in the bank.

But wait, there's more! How long until we can hit the reset button on our epigenomes, or zap those pesky senescent cells out of existence? A couple of decades? Maybe three? Who knows, but when those breakthroughs come knocking, they could add another glorious decade to our lifespan.

So, where does that leave us?

Drumroll, please... a conservative estimate of **113 years of life expectancy**!

That's right, folks, we're talking about living well into triple digits, with the potential for even more if we keep riding this wave of scientific innovation.

So, as we hurtle towards a future that's straight out of a sci-fi novel, remember this: for every month you manage to stay alive, you're earning yourself another precious week of life. Who knows, by the end of the century, you might just be adding a whole month to your lifespan every single month.

Now that's what I call a plot twist worth sticking around for!

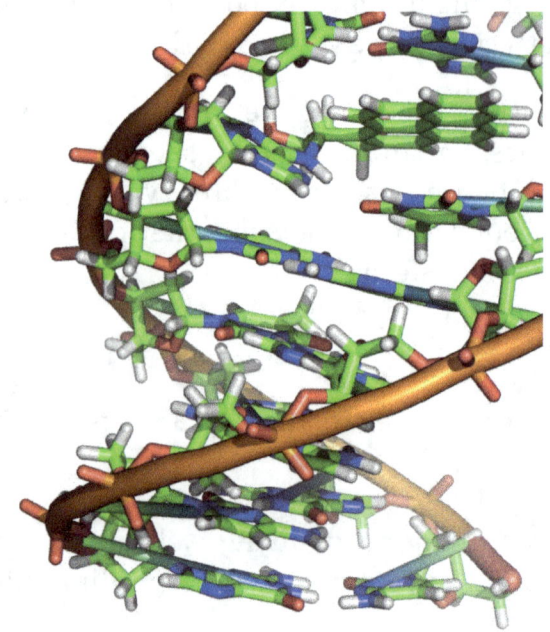

113 years of life expectancy

Alright, youngsters, gather around for a mind-boggling adventure through the land of numbers and possibilities!

We're about to decode some serious science talk into language even your pet goldfish can understand. Strap in, 'cause it's gonna be a wild ride!

So, imagine Jeanne Calment, the reigning champ of longevity, slowly slipping down the top-ten list of oldest humans in history.

It's like watching your favorite superhero lose their powers but with more candles on the cake. And guess what? It won't be long before she's out of the top 100, then the top million! Poof, just like that!

But hold onto your socks, 'cause here's where it gets juicy.

What if all those super cool technologies we're cooking up in labs could push the limits even further?

Picture this: people zipping past 110, 120, even 130 like it's no big deal! Could it happen? Maybe. But hey, no guarantees, just lots of wishful thinking.

Now, let's talk about scientists. These brainiacs are like superheroes with lab coats, and some of them are as optimistic as a puppy with a new chew toy.

They're cooking up potions to keep us kicking for longer, and they're not keeping it a secret anymore. Nope, they're shouting it from the rooftops like, "Hey, world, check out what we can do!"

But wait, there's more!

Even big-shot politicians, business folks, and the wise elders of society are starting to take notice. They're chatting about the future like it's the latest gossip, and let me tell ya, it's got 'em all fired up! They're brainstorming about how to handle a world where folks just keep on living and living.

Now, I could be wrong.

Yeah, I said it. But hey, life's full of surprises, right?

Just ask Albert Michelson, who thought he'd measured everything there was to measure, only to have quantum mechanics crash his party. Or Bill Gates, who missed the boat on the internet in his first draft of the future. Oops!

But here's the thing, youngsters: no matter what, we're in for a wild ride.

Our life spans are getting longer, and that means big changes ahead. So, let's buckle up and enjoy the journey, 'cause who knows what amazing discoveries await us?

As for me, I'll be here, soaking up every moment – whether I'm right or wrong, it's gonna be one heck of a ride!

Alright, folks, let's break down some mind-boggling numbers and explore the wacky world of future aging – with a sprinkle of humor, of course!

So, picture this: scientists are cooking up all sorts of crazy treatments that could potentially make us live longer than a tortoise's memoirs.

Some reckon that half of Japan's kiddos might hit a ripe old age of 107, while in the US, they're aiming for 104. That's like living long enough to see hoverboards become a reality – fingers crossed!

Now, some eggheads think those estimates are as inflated as a balloon at a birthday party, but not me. Nah, I'm tossing optimism around like confetti at a parade!

I'm talking about folks living to 100 and still kicking it like they're in their prime. And get this – 120 might just be the new 80! But hey, why stop there?

I'm boldly predicting that we'll soon be rubbing shoulders with the world's first-ever 150-year-old! Imagine the birthday cake for that bash!

But hold onto your hats, 'cause here's where things get a bit spooky. Some folks are freaking out like they've seen a ghost at a haunted house.

They're all like, "Whoa, hold up! If we start living forever, won't we just wreck the planet even more?" It's like realizing you've accidentally hit the fast-forward button on a disaster movie.

Now, I'm not just dodging these concerns like a ninja avoiding raindrops. Oh no, I'm listening, I'm nodding, I'm doing the whole "Hmm, interesting" routine.

But deep down, I'm still optimistic. I mean, come on, who wouldn't want more time for pizza parties and laser tag?

So, strap in, folks! We're on a rollercoaster ride through the maze of future possibilities, and I, for one, am ready to see where it takes us.

Bring on the birthday candles and the futuristic gadgets – the future's looking brighter than a neon sign on a sunny day!

Wasteful Mother Earth Warning!

Once upon a time, humans were like slow-cooking stew. We simmered for hundreds of thousands of years, but boy, were we close to getting burned to a crisp!

Back then, being over 40 was like finding a unicorn—super rare! Teenagers were playing grown-up games, being moms and warriors!

Life was like a fast-food drive-thru—order up, next, please! Only the speedy, brainy, brawny, and tough cookies made it. We got better at walking on two legs and thinking hard, but oof, it cost us a ton of lives and early checkouts.

Our ancestors were breeding like rabbits, just a hair quicker than they were kicking the bucket. But hey, it worked! We spread out all over the place, even before Columbus got lost.

Fast forward to now, and it's like squeezing into an elevator with way too many people. We're bumping elbows, heading for a cosmic game of sardines.

How many humans are too many?

Scientists say the Earth's party can handle about 8 billion guests. We're pretty much there now, and unless we're hoping for a zombie apocalypse or a "germs gone wild" party (which no sane person wants), the numbers won't stop growing.

Remember Frank Fenner, the guy who high-fived the eradication of smallpox? Well, he wasn't high fiving for long.

Retirement was too quiet for him; his brain just kept churning. For 20 years, he was like a broken record, warning about the human population explosion and our love affair with stuff.

He dropped his mic in 2010, saying we've hit the snooze button too many times. We're on a one-way train to extinction, folks!

But wait, there's more!

Back in the day, Thomas Malthus was ringing the dinner bell of doom, warning us that too many mouths would lead to too little food.

Then came Paul and Anne Ehrlich, shaking their population bomb like a baby rattle. Their book had a cover scarier than a ghost story—a chubby baby sitting on a ticking bomb. Cue the nightmares!

Inside, they painted a picture scarier than a haunted house: streets packed tighter than a can of sardines, with people doing everything from eating to... well, you name it!

Every year, the Ehrlich said, we're falling behind on food production, and our bellies are grumbling louder. While their crystal ball wasn't perfect (thank goodness!), they might have underestimated the real monster under our beds—a planet-sized temper tantrum that could wipe us all out!

Fast forward to 2016, and Stephen Hawking threw his two cents in, saying we've got about as much time left as a mayfly at a barbecue.
Humanities got a century to find a new place to crash, he said, because Earth's running out of room. Too bad the closest cosmic Airbnb is light-years away, and we're stuck with a horse-and-buggy spaceship!

So buckle up, folks! It's a wild ride to the future, and it's gonna be one heck of a rollercoaster!

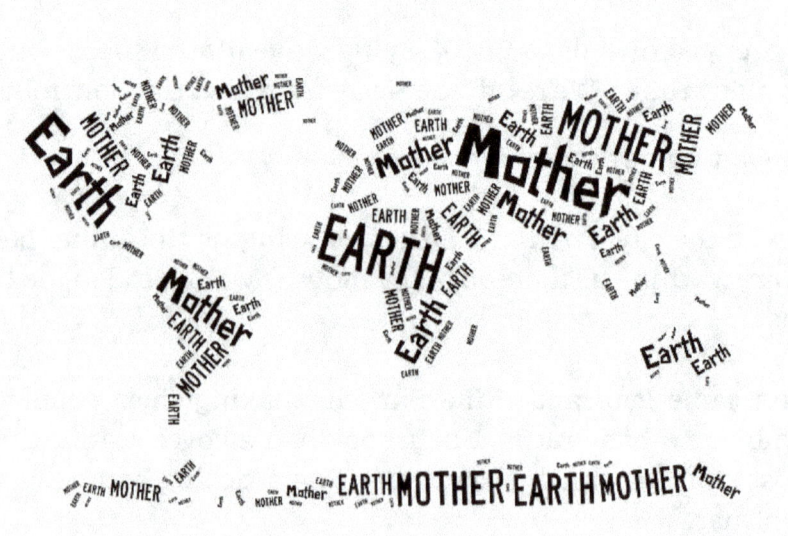

◆ ◆ ◆

Survival of the Funniest

Welcome to the "Survival of the Funniest: The Hundred Years' Comedy Hour"! Get ready to laugh your way through the impending doom of our planet.

So, picture this: Americans are like those folks at an all-you-can-eat buffet who fill their plates to the brim, only to leave half of it untouched and then dump the rest in the trash.

Seriously, they consume enough to feed a small army and produce more garbage than you can shake a stick at. And don't even get me started on their love affair with fossil fuels and plastic – it's like they're trying to win an award for the biggest carbon footprint.

But wait, it's not just Americans!

It's like a worldwide competition to see who can consume and waste the most. If everyone on Earth lived like Americans for just a year, we'd need a four-year timeout for the planet to recover.

Talk about unsustainable living – we're treating Earth like a rental car at a bachelor party.

And those scientists with their hundred-year warnings?

They're like the doomsday prophets of the modern era, except instead of shouting from street corners, they're publishing papers. They're telling us that even if we tried to clean up our act, we've already hit the point of no return. It's like trying to unbake a cake – not gonna happen.

But hey, it's not all bad news.

We're witnessing nature's great disappearing act – species going extinct faster than you can say "Oops, we did it again."

Coral reefs are turning white faster than an embarrassed ghost, and even cute little **marsupials** are going extinct because their homes are underwater. Talk about a tough housing market!

And if you live in a coastal city, you might want to invest in a snorkel because sea levels are rising faster than your uncle's cholesterol after Thanksgiving dinner.

Pretty soon, we'll all be living in Atlantis, except without the cool underwater architecture.

But hey, at least we'll have longer lifespans to enjoy the show, right? Wrong.
Turns out, the longer we stick around, the worse things get. It's like a never-ending sitcom with no laugh track.

So, buckle up, folks, because it's going to be a bumpy ride.

And remember, when life gives you climate change, make jokes – it's the only way we'll survive the hundred years' warning!

Climate Crisis Comedy Hour- Social Injustice

Ah, the Great Depression of the 1930s – a time when even your grandma and grandpa were feeling the financial pinch harder than a pair of too-tight shoes.

Stock markets crashing, banks tanking, and older folks watching their life savings swirl down the drain like water in a broken bathtub. It was a mess, folks.

Picture this: your kindly neighbor who used to bake the best apple pie in town, suddenly scraping by, wondering how they'll put food on the table. These were the days when desperation was as common as pigeons in the park, and the U.S. government had to step in with social security like a superhero in shiny armor.

Now, back then, hitting 65 was like reaching the golden age of bingo nights and early bird specials. You'd get a little extra cash to ease into those twilight years.

But here's the kicker: the number of folks living long enough to collect was smaller than a two-person parade, and the working crowd was footing the bill. It was like having 41 generous relatives willing to cover your tab at the diner.

Fast forward to today, where hitting 65 is as common as finding a Starbucks on every corner. People are retiring earlier, and living longer, and the ratio of workers to retirees is as wonky as a three-legged race.

Politicians? Oh, they love to dance around the issue like it's a hot potato.

Social Security? More like the third rail of politics – touch it, and you're toast. And with more and more seniors hitting the voting booths, they've got the political clout of a heavyweight champ.

But let's talk turkey here. The American Association of Retired Persons (AARP) isn't keen on changing the retirement game.

Sure, some folks might enjoy working longer, but spare a thought for those who've busted their backs in manual labor jobs. Asking them to clock in for another round is like sending a marathon runner back to the starting line after they've already crossed the finish.

And don't even get me started on the economic crystal ball-gazers.
Will people keep working?
Will robots take over the world before we retire?
Will we spend our golden years cruising the Caribbean or counting pennies like Scrooge McDuck?
Nobody knows, folks. We're as clueless as a cat in a yarn factory.

So buckle up, buttercups. We're hurtling into a retirement revolution faster than a granny at a Black Friday sale.

And while we may not have all the answers, one thing's for sure – it's going to be one heck of a ride!

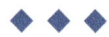

Riches and Wrinkles Forever

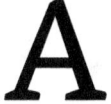Ah, the saga of wealth and longevity, where the rich seem to have found the fountain of youth while the rest of us are stuck with a leaky faucet.

Back in the '70s, being well-off not only meant having fancier cars and bigger houses but also an extra slice of life, roughly 1.2 years more than the folks scraping by.

Fast forward to today, and it's like the rich have discovered a cheating code for life.

While we mere mortals are busy worrying about bills, they're adding years to their existence like it's some kind of VIP club membership. It's not just about having a healthier lifestyle; it's about having a whole entourage of experts—doctors, trainers, nutritionists—making sure they're ticking for longer.

And let's not forget their penchant for dabbling in politics. Turns out, the tax code has been given more facelifts than a Hollywood starlet, all in favor of the well-heeled.

Estate taxes, originally meant to finance wars, now seem more like a 'rich person rebate' scheme, with loopholes big enough to drive a yacht through.

Meanwhile, the rest of us are left wondering if we'll ever see a tax break that doesn't involve rummaging through the couch cushions for spare change.

But hey, it's not all bad news.

While the wealthy are busy hoarding their riches and adding

zeros to their lifespans, the rest of us can take solace in the fact that aging still isn't considered a disease.

So, until the powers that be decide that wrinkles are a public health crisis, we'll just have to watch from the sidelines as the elite sip from the fountain of youth.

In the meantime, if you need me, I'll be over here trying to make my avocado toast last longer than my savings account.

Cheers to longevity, or at least to laughing through the wrinkles!

Rich vs Poor

Picture a world where the haves and have-nots are as divided as cats and dogs at a buffet table: a world where the privileged few, by some cosmic joke of fate, get to hang around for an extra three decades compared to the poor souls who can barely afford a decent pair of socks, let alone the latest longevity treatments promising to keep them sprightly.

We're tiptoeing into a future straight out of a sci-fi flick, where movies like Gattaca start to look less like entertainment and more like documentaries on how to breed superhumans.

Soon enough, gene editing will be as common as ordering takeout, with parents customizing their youngsters like a designer handbag. "Oh, I'll take the 'athletic prowess' option with a side of 'genius intellect,' please!"

And let's not forget our furry friends in this brave new world. If the rich can bankroll their own children's immortality, you can bet your bottom dollar they'll be lining up to extend the lives of their precious pets too. Fluffy the cat might just outlive us all.

But hold onto your hats, folks, because things could get wilder than a rodeo on Mars. If we don't start singing the equality tune, we're barreling toward a future where the gap between the wealthy and the rest of us isn't just about bank balances—it's about who gets to play God with life itself.

So, while we're busy debating whether to invest in the latest fad diet or just embrace our dad bods, let's not forget that our planet's resources aren't exactly limitless.

As biologist Edward O. Wilson once said, Earth's like a party hostess trying to keep the canapés coming with an ever-growing guest list.

And with billions more mouths to feed, we're starting to run out of snacks.

Mother Nature

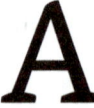h, the endless debate about the capacity of our dear old planet Earth to host our ever-expanding human circus.

Scientists, those noble warriors of evidence, like to think they're above the fray, scoffing at anything as pedestrian as "obviousness."

After all, it's not about what should be, it's about what the data says—unless, of course, you're debating whether pineapple belongs on pizza.

But hold onto your lab coats, folks, because we've got a renegade in our midst!

Enter Erle C. Ellis, the environmental scientist with a flair for stirring the pot. While others are busy wringing their hands over global limits, Ellis is out here throwing scientific shade like it's confetti at a birthday party.

Forget about traditional models, says Ellis. They're as outdated as a flip phone at a tech conference. According to him, our planet's capacity isn't some fixed number stamped on a cosmic ruler—it's a fluid concept, shaped by our ever-evolving social systems and the ingenuity of our technologies.

Cue the mic drop.

And let's not forget Ellis's bold proclamation in the hallowed halls of the New York Times: the idea of a global carrying capacity is about as sensible as a fish riding a bicycle.

Humans, he declares, have been thumbing their noses at so-called "natural limits" since the days when cavemen were busy inventing the wheel and arguing over the best way to cook a mammoth steak.

"We're niche creators!" Ellis cries, waving his PowerPoint clicker like a battle flag. "We bend ecosystems to our will, like a cosmic landscaper with a green thumb and a subscription to Popular Science."

So next time someone tries to tell you that humans need to play by Mother Nature's rulebook, just remember we've been rewriting the rules since we first picked up a stick and decided to call it a tool.

Who needs "natural" when you've got Wi-Fi, am I right?

We've come a long way since Thomas Hobbes penned his thoughts on life being a perpetual nightmare of "no arts; no letters; no society." Frankly, if that's what nature intended, count me out—I'd rather not live in a world where every day feels like a scene from a horror movie directed by Mother Nature herself.

And I'm willing to bet you're not signing up for that ride either.

So what is natural, you ask?

Well, sure, our primal instincts drive us to seek lives with fewer monsters under the bed and fewer wild swings from the saber-toothed tiger.

But let's not forget our knack for picking up cool tricks along the way, like chimps using sticks to score some tasty termite snacks or birds dropping rocks on stubborn shellfish like tiny avian barbarians.

Humans are like the MacGyvers of the animal kingdom, always finding new ways to MacGyver our way out of sticky situations.

Take the scientific method, for example—a brilliant invention that's propelled us from caveman-banging rocks together to the era of smartphones and avocado toast.

And don't even get me started on all the other goodies we've cooked up: cars, planes, laptops, TikTok dances—you name it, we've probably made it. Heck, even our pets living the high life in our cozy homes are part of the natural order of things.

But here's the kicker: the only thing truly unnatural in our story is the idea of sitting back and twiddling our opposable thumbs while the world passes us by.

We're wired to break boundaries, to push limits, and to always be on the lookout for the next big thing. And if that means tinkering with the fabric of time and space to squeeze a few more years out of this wild ride we call life, then pass me the spanner—I'm all in.

Sure, there are challenges ahead, like figuring out how to feed, clothe, and entertain billions more humans without turning the planet into a giant, overcrowded Chuck E. Cheese.

But hey, if there's one thing we humans excel at, it's finding creative solutions to our messes. Just look at our track record—the past century alone is a highlight reel of triumph over adversity.

So, can we do it?

Can we keep this crazy train chugging along without derailing into an apocalyptic hellscape? You bet your sweet bippy we can.

After all, if there's one thing we've learned from history, it's that when humanity puts its mind to something, there's no stopping us—except maybe for a bathroom break or two.

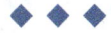

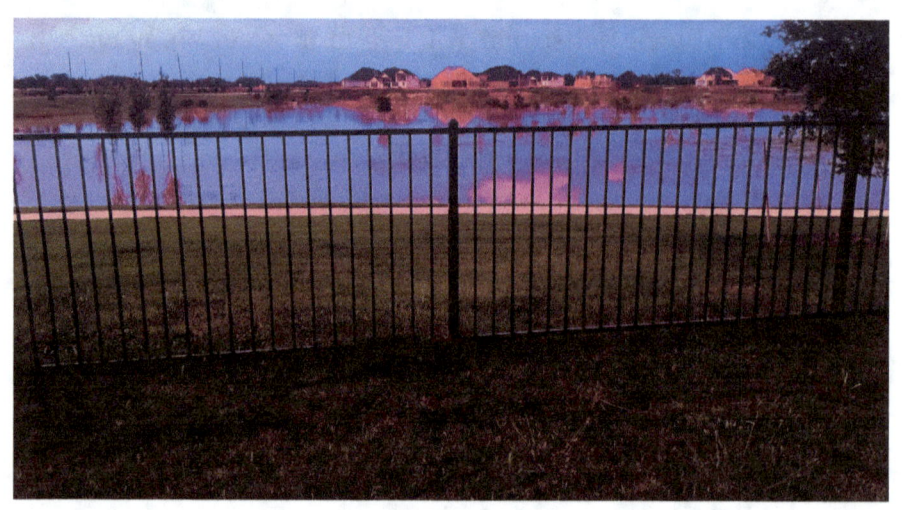

CHAPTER 2

People Overflow, Birth Control

Ah, the marvels of human population growth! From nearly biting the dust millennia ago to becoming the dominant species on this big blue marble, we've certainly come a long way.

It's like we're playing a game of "How Many People Can We Fit on Earth?" and we're winning... or are we?

Picture this: we're cramming ourselves into every nook and cranny of this planet at a rate that would make sardines jealous.

From **1 billion to 7.7 billion** in just a few blinks of the cosmic eye, we're practically breeding faster than rabbits at a disco.

But fear not, dear Earthlings, for the tides of population growth are turning. Thanks to the marvels of modernity—better opportunities for women, basic human rights (what a concept!), and the occasional bout of common sense—our population explosion is fizzling out like a damp firework.

Sure, we might've once thought death was our best bet for population control but turns out it's not that big of a deal.

Even if we hit pause overall "kicking the bucket" thing, we'd barely be making a dent in the human swarm. We're talking 55 million newbies a year, which, in the grand scheme of things, is like a drop in the ocean.

And hey, with all this talk about living longer and healthier, who knows? Maybe your great-great-grandma will be rocking her 150th birthday like it's nobody's business.

The sky's the limit... or rather, there is no limit! Who says we must punch out at a certain age anyway?

So, while some folks might still be fretting over the specter of overpopulation, we're just here, living our best lives, one human at a time. After all, it's not the end of the world... yet.

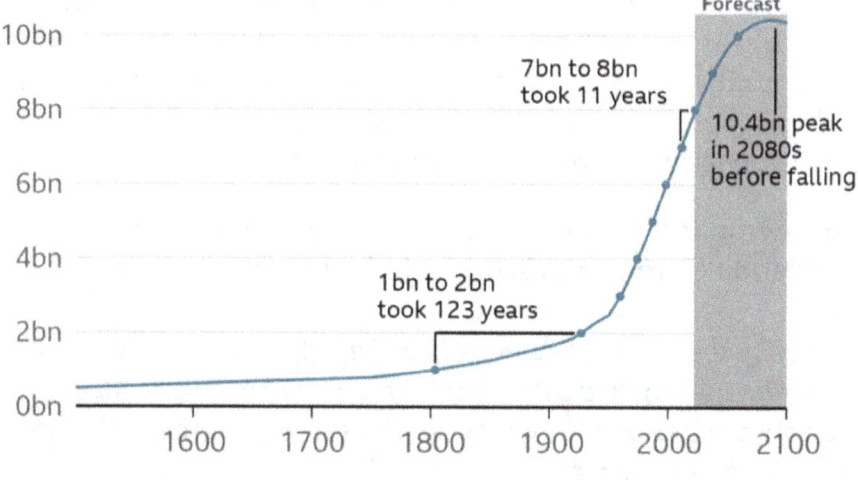

Eastern vs Western Alliances

A h, the slow march of progress! We might be pushing the boundaries of our expiration dates, but let's not get ahead of ourselves.

Death's not throwing in the towel just yet, folks. We're still on a first-name basis with the Grim Reaper, and it seems like we'll be keeping that acquaintance for a while longer.

But fear not, for amidst this dance with mortality, there's a glimmer of hope—or at least a slightly less frenetic pace of procreation.

Birth rates have been plummeting like a skydiver without a

parachute, so while we might still be adding more heads to the human pyramid, it's more like a leisurely stroll than a sprint.

Instead of quaking in our boots at the thought of a more modest population bump, let's throw a party for survival!

I mean, come on, folks, we didn't just survive the past century of explosive growth—we practically aced it! Sure, we may have left a trail of destruction in our wake and cooked up some rather unsavory deeds along the way, but hey, we're still here, right?

Now, let's talk optimism—or rather, the lack thereof.

Turns out, when asked whether the world's getting better or worse, folks in the Western world are about as cheery as a wilted daisy. In the good ol' U.S. of A., only a measly 6 percent are popping champagne for global progress. And that's the optimistic bunch!

But hold your horses, because in the rest of the world, things aren't nearly as gloomy. Nope, elsewhere, people are more optimistic than a kid with a lemonade stand on a hot summer's day.

Sure, we've had our fair share of hiccups—economic downturns, historical baggage, and enough bad news to fill a library—but let's not lose sight of the bigger picture.

The future's still out there, folks, and it's looking brighter than a neon sign in Times Square. So chin up, buttercups, and let's march forward with a smile on our faces and a skip in our step.

The world's not surprising us yet!

Picture this: in China, a land so vast it could probably fit a hundred world wonders, a bunch of folks were asked about the future.

Turns out, 80% of them were like, "Hey, the next generation's gonna have it better than us!" Talk about confidence!

And it's not just China, oh no!

Brazil, Russia, India, Turkey—these places are all saying, "Yeah, life's getting better!"

Sure, they're splurging a bit more on stuff, but they're also bringing down the baby-making rates, kicking poverty to the curb, and getting cozy with clean water and electricity. It's like the world's getting an upgrade, one country at a time!

But hold onto your hats, 'cause here comes the plot twist turns out, that being a downer is often a sign of being super-duper lucky.

Yup, when you look at the big picture, it's kind of hard to argue that the world's going down the drain. Nope, not when extreme poverty has been getting a serious beatdown, and more people than ever are trading in their dunce caps for diplomas.

I mean, think about it: two hundred years ago, it was like poverty was everyone's favorite accessory. But now? Extreme poverty is just a fading trend, like parachute pants or disco.

And don't even get me started on literacy rates! Back in the day, being able to read was as rare as finding a unicorn. But now? Four out of five people can read, and they've got Google at their fingertips!

Now, let's talk about why all this good stuff's happening.

Is it 'cause we're multiplying like rabbits on a hot date? Maybe.

But honestly, who cares? The point is, the world's getting better, and it's not because we're all competing to see who can pop out the most babies.

So, here's the deal: more people, longer lives, and a whole lot of improvements. And you know what? We've got our elders to thank for a big chunk of it! Sure, they might be battling a bunch of health issues, but they've still got the brains to run circles around us young'uns.

So, there you have it, folks: the world's getting better, and it's all thanks to a little thing called progress.

So, let's keep on dreaming big and making the world a better place—one laugh, one lesson, and one elder at a time!

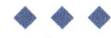

Saga of Retirement

Alright, buckle up for a wild ride through the world of work and retirement! So, imagine this: you're getting older, but instead of packing up your desk and heading for the golf course, you decide to stick around a bit longer.

And guess what? That's cool!

See, the longer we keep folks healthy and kickin', the more bang we get for our buck. It's like when you buy a bag of chips and find extra ones at the bottom—score!

But hey, just 'cause you can work longer doesn't mean you have to. Once you've paid your dues to society and can take care of yourself, why not do whatever floats your boat?

Now, some folks worry that if nobody retires, there won't be enough jobs for the young'uns. But let me tell you, that's like worrying you'll run out of pizza at a party. There's plenty to go around! Countries with older retirement ages tend to have a bigger economic pie to share.

Remember those old-timey fears about machines stealing everyone's jobs?

Turns out, they were about as accurate as a fortune teller with a magic eight ball. Sure, things change, but that doesn't mean we're all going to be out of work. Just look at how many women joined the workforce over the years—it didn't mean men lost their jobs, did it?

And get this: keeping folks in the game longer might save our bacon when it comes to stuff like Social Security. Instead of forcing folks to punch the clock 'til they drop, we should give them the choice.

And trust me, with all the perks that come with staying healthy and working, a lot of folks will want to stick around.

So, let's flip the script on retirement and embrace a future where folks keep on trucking' well into their golden years.

Who knows, maybe I'll still be cracking jokes in the lab at 80, surrounded by a crew of young whippersnappers eager to change the world.

And hey, with a bit of luck and some science magic, I might not even look a day over 50!

◆ ◆ ◆

Epic: Defeat Aging!

Behold! The Epic Saga of Dana Goldman and the Quest to Defeat Aging!

Once upon a time in the land of economics, Dana Goldman stood amidst a torrent of naysayers, like a lone hero facing an army of pessimists armed with spreadsheets.

They cried out about the swelling costs of healthcare, the impending doom of Social Security, and the nightmare of billions growing old simultaneously, creating an economic maelstrom of catastrophic proportions.

But lo and behold!

Goldman, with the wisdom of an economist and the spirit of a warrior, saw a glimmer of hope amidst the chaos.

What if, he pondered, we could not just extend lives, but extend healthy lives?

For in the realm of aging, every wrinkle comes with a hefty price tag, draining both wallets and society's vitality.

And so, armed with nothing but numbers and a trusty calculator, Goldman embarked on a daring journey to crunch the data.

His quest led him to a revelation: tackling one disease at a time was like playing an eternal game of medical whack-a-mole.

But delaying aging itself? Now that was the golden ticket! With aging delayed, diseases would tremble, and healthcare costs would cower in fear.

Imagine a world where treatments cost mere pennies, where families spent their final days together instead of in sterile hospital rooms, and where the phrase "aging in place" became as outdated as dial-up internet.

The peace dividend from this battle against aging would be vast, a treasure trove of trillions that could fund a new age of discovery.

But Goldman's vision didn't stop there. He dreamed of a world where women had more time for both career and parenting, where age discrimination was banished, and where retirees rejoined the workforce with gusto, armed with wisdom and experience.

Picture it: a workforce bustling with septuagenarian superheroes, armed not with canes but with knowledge and determination.

With each passing year, society would grow stronger, wiser, and more resilient, tackling challenges like climate change and education with renewed vigor.

And so, dear reader, let us join Dana Goldman on his quest to unleash the storm of the sickest - not with swords and shields, but with data and determination.

For in the battle against aging, the greatest weapon of all is the indomitable human spirit.

Age Defiance- Future Potential

Aging Defiance: Future Possibilities, Once upon a time in the groovy 70s, two brainiacs had a wild idea: let's test out that Bible tale about the Good Samaritan.

You know, the one where a dude helps another dude in a jam.

So, they set up this hilarious scenario at a seminary. They hired a fake dude to act like he was dying next to a building, and they roped in a bunch of seminary students to see what they'd do.

But here's the twist: they told some of the students they had all the time in the world, others they were running late, and the rest they had to dash like they were on fire to get to their talk.

Guess what?

The ones who were in a mad rush barely stopped to give the poor fake dude a high five, let alone help him up.

Meanwhile, the chill ones strolling along were like, "Yo, dude, need a hand?" It wasn't about being good or holy; it was all about feeling late for a hot date with destiny.

This is not exactly breaking news. Even back in ancient Rome, this dude Seneca was saying, "Hey, slow down, smell the roses, life's too short to be stressful." He was all about taking it easy, not freaking out about the past or sweating about the future.

So, here's the kicker: when we have more time, we're more likely to be decent human beings. Imagine if we had centuries to live instead of just decades. We might stop and think before doing something dumb.

But let's be real, even with all that time, we might still goof around. Time flies when you're having fun, right?

So, the real question is, how do we want to spend all that time?

Do we want to party 'til the sun burns out, or do we want to team up and build a world that doesn't suck?

The choices we make now will decide whether we end up in a sci-fi disaster flick or a utopian paradise.

And trust me, preventing diseases and keeping ourselves healthy is key to avoiding a total mess caused by climate change and other drama.

So yeah, buckle up, folks.

We might be living way longer than we ever thought possible. Who knows, maybe someday celebrating your 150th birthday will be as normal as eating cake.
And if that sounds far-fetched, just remember, some smarty-pants think half of today's youngsters will party like it's 2124.

Now that's what I call futureproofing!

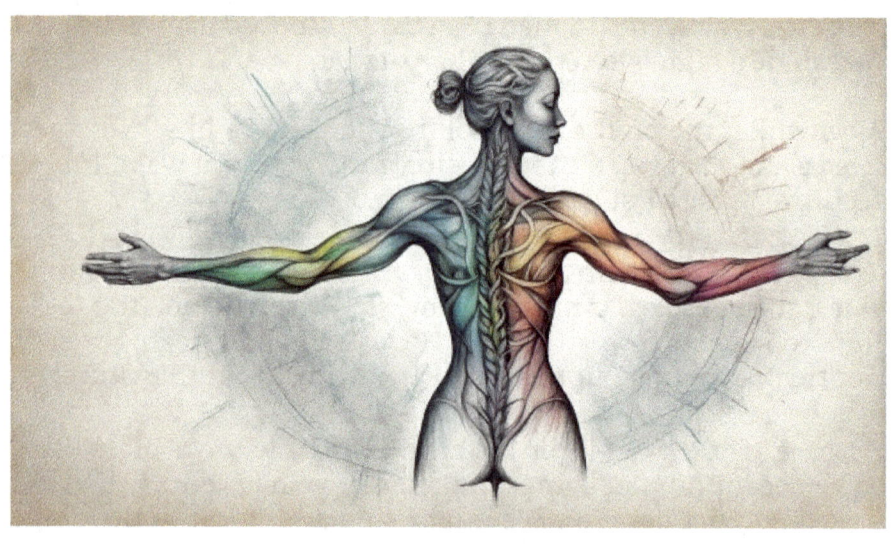

◆ ◆ ◆

Alright, buckle up, folks!

For those skeptics out there who think this whole "defying

aging" thing is just a bunch of hogwash, let me enlighten you with a dose of reality!

Either you're clueless about science or you're playing ostrich with your head buried in the sand. Either way, you're likely to eat your words sooner than you think, especially with progress zooming along at warp speed. Who would've thought, huh?

Now, listen up!

There's no biological memo floating around saying we must kick the bucket at 80.

And guess what? No divine Post-it notes are decreeing we're done after hitting the big 80 either.

Heck, according to Genesis, Isaac was kicking it at the ripe old age of 180! Go figure!

Thanks to some nifty technologies I won't bore you with, a longer, healthier life is basically in the cards. The how's and when's are a tad fuzzy, but trust me, we're getting there.

With stuff like **AMPK** activators, **TOR** inhibitors, and **sirtuin** activators doing their thing, and a bunch of smart cookies in lab coats tinkering away, the odds are stacking up in our favor.

But wait, there's more! We're not just talking about slapping on a few extra years.

Oh no, we're talking about revving up our engines with Senolytics and cellular reprogramming, plus a sprinkle of personalized Tender Loving Care to keep our bodies ticking like Swiss watches.
And don't forget the little lifestyle tweaks we can all make to activate our longevity genes and snag some extra good years.

So, here's the kicker: What kind of world do you want to live in?

Are you cool with a future where the rich keep getting richer and outlive us all? Or how about a dystopian nightmare where everyone's fighting over the last crumbs of resources while the planet melts like a popsicle on a hot summer day?

If that's your jam, then hey, sit back, grab some popcorn, and enjoy the show!

But hold on to your hats because there's another option on the menu!

Picture this: a world were staying forever young isn't just a pipe dream but a golden ticket to a brighter, greener, more kick-ass future for all.

Imagine a world where we're not just throwing cash at curing diseases but tackling global challenges head-on.

It's a world where the old-timers are the real MVPs, hailed for their wisdom and savvy. It's a world where being a Good Samaritan isn't just a nice gesture but a global norm.

Sounds awesome, right? Well, here's the catch: It isn't going to happen on its own.
We got to roll up our sleeves and get to work, folks! So, who's with me? Let's make tomorrow's headlines today!

Funding for Research

Alright, picture this: I'm an entrepreneur physician, all about innovation, and super grateful for folks investing in solving tough problems.

But here's the thing: the market doesn't automatically churn out groundbreaking science or fair healthcare solutions. We need a mix of public and private cash to fuel research, spark discoveries, and make sure everyone benefits.

Recently, this balance has been off kilter. Since 2017, the US government hasn't been the main funder of basic science like it used to be.

It all started back in the late 1800s when the government began funding scientific research, but nowadays, there's less certainty about that funding.

The National Institutes of Health (NIH), for instance, gets its funding from Congress, and it's been a lifeline for countless medical breakthroughs.
Without NIH money, we wouldn't have many of the meds and treatments we rely on today.

Sure, the government still kicks in a lot of dough for medical research, which is great because it means scientists can chase our wild ideas without worrying too much about making a quick buck.

But with funding getting tighter, scientists studying aging – a big deal are turning more to private backers.

Alright, buckle up for a ride through the wacky world of research funding, especially when it comes to aging.

Picture this: scientists trying to figure out how to keep us all spry and healthy for longer are struggling to get the cash they need.

So, here's the scoop: despite more and more people getting older and healthcare costs skyrocketing, the money going into understanding aging biology is less than a drop in the ocean of medical research funds.

Why, you ask? Well, it's like this global game of "definition by disease" that ties up funding.

If you're a smarty-pants scientist with a brilliant idea to tackle cancer or Alzheimer's, you're in luck. Big bucks are waiting for you from places like the NIH. They're like the fairy godmother of medical research, handing out grants left and right.
But when it comes to aging, it's like trying to get blood from a stone.

Let's break down the numbers, shall we?

Heart disease gets a hefty $1.7 billion, Cancer's rolling in with $6.3 billion, and Alzheimer's gets a cool $3 billion.

But how about Obesity, which affects a whopping 30% of the population and shaves off years of life? Less than a billion. Yep, you read that right.

Now, before you start imagining a world without your beloved coffee, consider this: the government's spending on aging research in 2018 was chump change compared to what we splurge on Java every year.

And let's be real, life without coffee? No thanks. But if you're a scientist wanting to crack the code of aging, it's like hitting a brick wall.

In 2018, Congress chucked a measly $3.5 billion towards aging research.

But guess what? Almost all of it went towards studying Alzheimer's, running tests on hormone therapies, and checking out how old folks live. Less than 3% went into understanding the nitty-gritty of **aging** biology.

Here's the kicker: aging messes with 93% of folks over 50, yet the NIH is throwing peanuts at it compared to the cash they shower on cancer research.
It's like the scientific equivalent of giving a kid a dime when they ask for a dollar.

So yeah, the struggle is real for aging researchers, my friends.

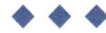

Alright, let's dive into the wild world of science funding and aging with Leonard Hayflick, the brainiac who discovered something called the Hayflick Limit.

He's a bit miffed that the big bucks seem to be flowing into specific diseases like Alzheimer's, leaving other aspects of aging high and dry.

Hayflick points out that curing Alzheimer's might only give us an extra 19 days of life, which, let's face it, is hardly enough time to binge-watch your favorite show.

He's not saying we should ditch Alzheimer's research altogether – he's just annoyed that it doesn't help us understand aging.

Now, compared to other countries, the US throws a decent chunk of change into aging research. But here's the kicker: nobody officially calls aging a disease.

Yep, you read that right. Even though it's the granddaddy of all diseases, it doesn't get the same treatment as, say, heart disease or cancer.

Hayflick reckons if we start treating aging like the sneaky disease it is, it could revolutionize research. Suddenly, labs everywhere would be buzzing with scientists trying to crack the aging code.

And let me tell you, there are plenty of eager young minds itching to get in on the action.

The first country to officially label aging as a disease could be onto something big. Think jobs, innovation, and a whole lot of bragging rights. And hey, who wouldn't want to be known as the nation that put aging in its place?

But hey, let's not forget about the ethical side of all this.

With great scientific power comes great responsibility, right? We got to make sure we're using these breakthroughs for the greater good and not turning ourselves into superhumans without a second thought.

So, in a nutshell, it's time to give aging the respect it deserves in the world of science.

Because who knows, maybe the key to a longer, healthier life is just waiting to be discovered – and it's about time we gave it the attention it needs.

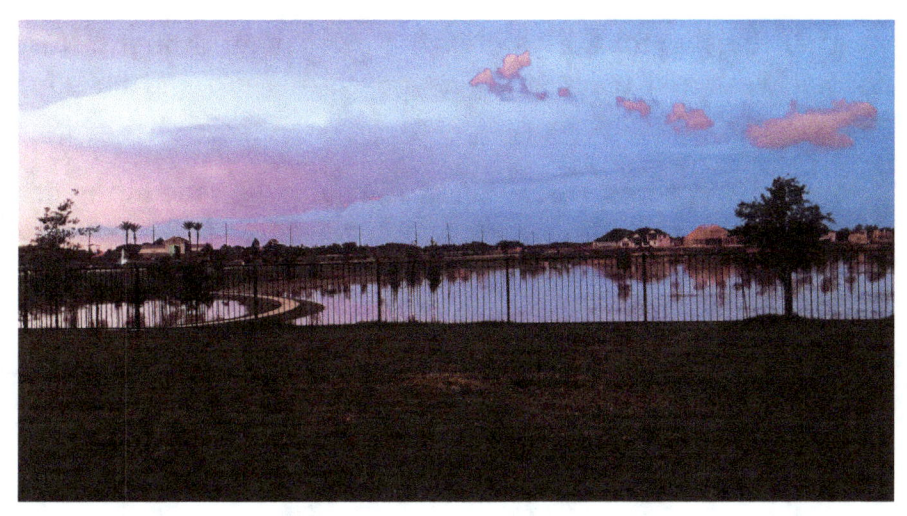

CHAPTER 3

Fix Senior's Tooth Trouble

Alright, buckle up for a wild ride through the Bill of Rights - the dental edition!

So, there I was, reclining in the dentist's chair, feeling like a contestant on a toothy game show. The dentist, with all the enthusiasm of a librarian on a slow Thursday afternoon, peered into my mouth.

"Your teeth are fine," she proclaimed as if announcing the

weather forecast for a region with a permanent drought. "Just normal wear and tear. Let's get you cleaned up and on your merry way."

Before I could protest, she was already mentally scheduling her next coffee break. But I wasn't about to let this tooth travesty slide.

"Doctor, hold up a sec," I interjected. "Could you elaborate on this 'normal wear and tear' business?"

She glanced at me, clearly unamused by my dental curiosity.

"Well, you're aging, and so are your teeth," she explained as if this were some profound revelations. "Your front teeth are wearing down naturally. If you were a teenager, we might do something about it, but—"

I cut her off. "Well, guess what? I want them fixed."

After some back-and-forth, the dentist reluctantly agreed, probably realizing that arguing with me was like trying to floss a hippo's teeth.

I may have dropped the fact that I planned to keep these chompers for a long, long time and that I wasn't afraid to break the bank for it.

But this dental saga isn't just about me and my gnashers; it's a snapshot of how we middle-aged folks are treated in the healthcare circus.
When you hit the big 50, doctors seem more interested in keeping you 'es sick' than ensuring you'll be dancing in your golden years. Who hasn't had a doctor mutter those dreaded words: "Well, you're not twenty anymore"?

In the medical world, age and money call the shots.

Most of my Doctors' colleague often shy away from discussing treatments that could keep us spry, assuming we're all destined for a slow slide into creaky old age.

And let's not forget the almighty dollar, which dictates who gets what treatment, regardless of how much it could improve our quality of life.

It's high time we ditched this ageist nonsense. Medical care shouldn't be discriminated based on wrinkles or bank balances. Whether you're pushing 90 or barely out of your twenties, you deserve the same level of care and attention.

And don't worry about the cash. By investing in preventive care rather than scrambling to fix problems later, we'll save trillions in the long run. It's a win-win for everyone.

So, let's rewrite the rules.
Let's ensure that everyone, regardless of their birth year, has access to treatments that make life a little brighter.

Because in a world where age is just a number, it's about time our healthcare system caught up.

Future of Healthcare

Many people worry that getting fair access to medical care might cost too much money.
That's because healthcare programs worldwide are struggling to afford treatments, especially for very sick, elderly folks who might only get a few extra years out of it.

But the future of healthcare shouldn't be all about treating diseases.

If we focus on helping people age well, we could tackle a big cause of illness. New drugs to keep us healthy as we get older could be super cheap compared to treating all the diseases they'd prevent.

A study from 2005 found that preventing diseases like diabetes or treating cancer costs a ton of money.

But investing in an "anti-aging" drug that could keep us healthy for an extra decade would be way cheaper. It's like spending a penny to save a dollar.

But what if these drugs just make us live longer without making us healthier?
That's like using medicine to make a car run longer without fixing what's broken. We need to talk about whether it's worth it to make people live longer if they're not going to feel better.

Luckily, it seems like these scary scenarios won't come true.

When we have good drugs to slow down aging, they'll also help us stay healthier longer. Then, healthcare will mostly be about easy stuff like check-ups and fixing emergencies, which is way cheaper than treating diseases.

It's a bit like switching from an old, high-maintenance car to a fancy electric one that hardly needs any fixing.

And while some countries are getting better at healthcare, others are lagging. Sadly, the United States is one of those falling behind.

Even though it spends a lot of money on healthcare, many people still can't get the care they need, which is pretty backward.

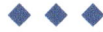

Alright, let's sprinkle some humor into this rant about medical mishaps and inequality!

So, I don't want to sound like I'm dissing the land of the free and the home of the brave—it's been pretty swell to me and my kin. But seriously, ever since I landed in the country that sent folks to the moon, I've been gobsmacked by how we manage to waste opportunities to help more people while spending less dough.

Now, the good old' US of A has been flexing its muscles in medical research, both with government dollars and private pocket change. It's like the nation's been throwing cash at labs like it's going out of style.

And you know what? We're cooking up drugs like nobody's business. We're responsible for churning out more meds than a hypochondriac's dream vacation.

But here's the kicker: while we're slaving away in our labs, making breakthroughs left and right, who's reaping the

benefits?
Not us Yanks, I'll tell you that much.
Nope, it's our pals across the pond, like the Brits, Swedes, Dutch, Irish, and even the Slovenians.

They're living it up with longer lifespans and healthier years thanks to their sweet universal healthcare setup.

Meanwhile, back in the good old US of A, we're arguing about who deserves what, waving our pitchforks at Capitol Hill like we're auditioning for a modern-day remake of "The Beverly Hillbillies."

Seriously, why aren't we demanding better healthcare, marching with signs that say, "More Meds, Less Madness"?

And don't even get me started on our politicians. They're out here claiming we've got the best healthcare system in the world like we're all living in some kind of medical utopia.

Newsflash: we're ranked lower than your average spring break destination by the World Health Organization!

It's like we're living in a world where the rich get to sip champagne on their yachts while the rest of us are drowning in medical bills. Talk about a divide bigger than the Grand Canyon!

But fear not, my friends! There's hope on the horizon.

If we can all get access to the fancy-pants technologies that keep us spry and healthy, maybe—just maybe—we can start closing the gap between the haves and the have-nots.

It's a small step for mankind, but a giant leap for equality!

Cosmic Lifespan and Euthanasia

Ah, the cosmic musings on life and death, brought to you by Pratika Dayal, the stargazing philosopher extraordinaire.

In this vast universe, where planets dance and stars twinkle, we find ourselves on this little blue marble, debating the ultimate question: Can we choose our exit strategy?

Picture this: giant elliptical galaxies, double the size of ours and overflowing with habitable planets like a cosmic Costco.

Yet here we are, stuck on this rock, with our closest potential vacation spot being a mere twelve light-years away. Sure, it sounds close until you realize it's like waiting for your Uber after a night out—only 10,000 years of sobering up required.

Meet our hypothetical neighbors from Maffei 1. These guys are so advanced that they probably think our moon landing was a quaint backyard barbecue.

They'd ask us the tough questions: Have we unlocked the secrets of the universe? Have we learned to use our resources without blowing ourselves up? Have we mastered the art of sustainable living?

Spoiler alert: We're still figuring out how to recycle without turning it into an extreme sport.

Then comes the awkward part where we show off our achievements, like sending a dozen dudes to the moon. "Where's

Luna?" they'd ask, and we'd point to our nightlight in the sky. Cue the cosmic facepalm.

But the real kicker comes when they ask about our lifespan. Have we cracked the code on living forever? "Uh, we just started thinking about it yesterday," we'd admit, hoping they're as forgiving as grandparents watching a toddler attempt to walk.

Now, onto the million-light-year question: How do we kick the bucket?

Brace yourselves, folks, because right now, it's not exactly a graceful exit. We're talking diseases crashing our life party like uninvited guests, making us suffer through a prolonged and agonizing farewell tour.

But fear is not, for science comes to the rescue! Turns out, the longer we keep rodents alive, the quicker they punch their tickets. It's like they're saying, "Enough is enough, I'm out here," and dropping the mic. We should take notes.

So, let's talk about "physician-assisted peace-out," or as I like to call it, "Choose Your Adventure: The Final Chapter."

It's time to ditch the archaic laws and give people the dignity to bid adieu on their terms, without playing cosmic hopscotch to find a peaceful exit. Because in the grand tapestry of the universe, shouldn't we have the right to bow out with a little grace and a lot less drama?

Imagine being in the shoes of David Goodall, an English-born Australian, a remarkable ecologist faced with an unimaginable dilemma at the age of 104.

He was forced to leave his home, where the compassionate

option of physician-assisted suicide is sadly prohibited, he embarked on a poignant journey to Switzerland, where such a choice is not only legal but also dignified.

No soul should ever have to confront the heart-wrenching decision of either expiring in a foreign land or, worse, ending their life as a criminal act on their final earthly breath.

In a world where wisdom and life experience are cherished, where the investment in education reaches its culmination around the age of 40, it is unjust to withhold the right to choose one's departure from those of sound mind.

And for those grappling with the relentless grip of terminal illness or chronic pain, regardless of age, compassion dictates that they should be afforded the same compassionate choice.

Rules are necessary, of course. Guidance and counseling are paramount, alongside a thoughtful waiting period. The decision to embrace one's final moments should never be taken lightly or impulsively, akin to facing the swirling tumult of adolescence. If it were that simple, many of us might not have weathered the storm of our teenage years.

Yet, let us not burden rational adults with guilt or shame for seeking control over their final chapter.

Every day, conversations unfold where individuals candidly express their reluctance to extend their journey beyond a certain point.

"If I reach a hundred, just put me out of my misery," they jest.

"Seventy-five healthy years sound just about right," they ponder.

And some, with a humorous glint, admit, "I can't fathom enduring my spouse's company any longer than I already have."

Indeed, the prospect of eternal existence holds little allure for many. Recently, I engaged with a diverse audience spanning generations, and their responses were telling.

Some were content with 80 years, others aspired to see 120, and a daring few envisioned stretching their journey to 150. Immortality, however, was a notion embraced by only a handful.

Similar sentiments echoed in discussions amongst esteemed scientists studying aging, where the pursuit of immortality found few champions.

Most who harbor such dreams aren't paralyzed by fear of death; rather, they harbor an unyielding love for life, their families, and their careers, and an insatiable curiosity for the unfolding future.

I, too, hold no fondness for death, not out of fear of the unknown, but from a place of profound appreciation for the precious gift of life.

When turbulence rattles the calm of an airplane cabin, my wife's grip tightens while my pulse remains steady. Having faced the specter of mortality in airborne mishaps, I've learned that letting go of fear was among the most liberating acts I've ever embraced.

Let's delve into the fascinating realm of human desires: when a survey revealed the tantalizing prospect of retaining boundless health regardless of age, the enthusiasm for eternal life skyrocketed. Suddenly, nearly everyone yearned for immortality.

But beneath this longing lies a deeper fear—not of losing life itself, but of losing the essence of what makes us human.

And it's a fear that strikes at the core of our humanity. I witnessed this firsthand through the suffering of my patients every night in the ICU of the hospital I work for, who endured years of illness before passing away in their early 70s.

Trapped in a vegetative state for what felt like an eternity, their heart, aided by a relentless pacemaker, stubbornly clung to life, albeit devoid of vitality. It's a harrowing fate—a life preserved, but devoid of health and dignity.

In my eyes, there are few cruelties as profound as prolonging life without preserving health. This distinction is paramount.

What good is an extended lifespan if it's marred by suffering? If we're to extend our years, we bear an undeniable moral obligation to ensure those years are lived in good health.

Like many, I'm not seeking an eternity; I simply yearn for a life abundant with wellness and love.

For those immersed in the quest against aging, it's not about defying death; it's about granting individuals the gift of more vibrant years, allowing them to face death on their terms—swiftly, peacefully, and when they're ready.

Whether it's by eschewing treatments that prolong life without quality or by embracing interventions while retaining the autonomy to depart when the time feels right, no one who has repaid their societal debt should feel tethered to this world against their will.

It's high time we embark on the journey of crafting cultural, ethical, and legal frameworks that honor this fundamental human right.

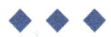

Innovative Solution for

Consumption and Waste

Alright, gather around, folks! It's time to tackle the big brown elephant in the room – human waste and consumption – but we're going to do it with a twist of humor and a sprinkle of innovation!

So, you've got George Monbiot, this environmental guru, shouting from the rooftops that we're all fussing over how many humans are crammed onto this spinning rock when really, it's our insatiable appetite for stuff that's doing all the damage.

George might be a bit of a lefty, but on this one, he's hitting the nail on the head – it's not the headcount, it's munching down on resources like they're an all-you-can-eat buffet at a Vegas casino.

Sure, we know humans can survive on a lot less – I mean, have you seen those minimalist influencers living in tiny houses?

But will we do it? That's the billion-dollar question.

Some scientists reckon we'll figure out how to stretch our resources like elastic, while others are betting on humanity's talent for gobbling up everything in sight until we're swimming in our garbage like a bunch of seagulls at a landfill picnic.

But fear not, my friends, because where there's a will, there's a way – and that way is paved with politics and technology. Take a gander at the "stuff factor" – technology's magic trick of making physical things disappear faster than a rabbit in a hat.

Remember when your room was stacked floor to ceiling with CDs and DVDs? Now, it's all about streaming and digital downloads.

Need a ride? Just summon a car with your phone – no need for your gas-guzzler.

Heck, even hospitals are ditching the paper trail for cloud-connected tablets faster than you can say "medical breakthrough."

So, let's raise a toast to the power of human ingenuity and a hearty belly laugh at our wasteful ways. With a little innovation and a whole lot of humor, maybe we can turn this ship around before it's too late.

Alright, buckle up, folks!

Steven Pinker, the guru of wit and wisdom, has cracked open the can of truth and spilled it everywhere – we're ditching the hoarding of "stuff" for cleaner air, safer rides, and drugs for diseases that even the germs don't remember.

And while we used to measure our wealth in square footage, now it's all about fitting our lives into apartments the size of shoeboxes and calling it chic.

Gone are the days of McMansions swallowing up the countryside like a hungry hippo. Nope, we're downsizing faster than your grandma's recipe for cookies.

We've traded in the manicured lawns for community spaces where you can sweat it out in the gym, gossip in the kitchen, and maybe even find love in the laundry room.

Talk about a living space where you're never alone – unless you're hiding from your neighbor's weird cat.

But hold your horses, folks! Just because we're shedding our love affair with things doesn't mean we've kicked all our bad habits.
Oh no, we're still chugging water like it's going out of style, tossing food like it's a hot potato, and burning through energy like it's going out of fashion.

According to the United Nations, we're making Mother Nature's job harder than a cat herding contest.

We're polluting water like it's our job, tossing out enough food to feed a small planet, and all the while, millions are left hungry and grumbling in their bellies.

And here's the kicker – by 2050, we'll be sucking the planet dry faster than a juice box at a toddler's birthday party.

But fear not, dear Earthlings, for technology is here to save the day!

We may not be able to force folks to stop gobbling up resources like they're at an all-you-can-eat buffet, but we can sure make it tempting to dial it back a notch.

So, let's raise a toast to smaller spaces, bigger hearts, and a future where we consume with a little less gusto and a whole lot more smarts.

After all, it's our planet, and it's the only one with chocolate.

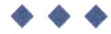

GMO Train

Listen up, folks! If we want to keep our bellies full and our planet happy, we got to get on board the GMO train.

Yeah, you heard me right – **genetically modified crops are the future of food**, and we better embrace them like we embrace our morning cup of coffee.

Now, I know what you're thinking – GMOs? Sounds scarier than a horror movie marathon on Halloween night.

But hold onto your pitchforks and torches, because these Franken crops are our ticket to feeding millions more hungry mouths without turning the Midwest into a giant salad bowl.

Sure, some folks out there are waving the "unnatural" flag like it's going out of style, but let's get real for a second – pretty much everything we munch on has been tinkered with more than your grandpa's old truck.

Take corn, for instance. That crunchy goodness you throw on the grill looks nothing like its wild ancestor, thanks to centuries of genetic makeovers that turned it into the juicy cob we know and love today.

And don't even get me started on apples – those little guys went from sour to sweet faster than a Kardashian's mood swings. So, next time you're munching on a crisp Granny Smith, just remember, nature had a little help from us meddling humans.

But hey, don't take my word for it – the big shots at the National

Academy of Sciences have given GMOs the green light, saying they're as safe as grandma's apple pie.

And let's face it, if you're more worried about GMOs than climate change, you might want to check your priorities. I mean, we've got more studies backing up GMO safety than there are TikTok videos of cats doing weird stuff.

So, let's put aside the fearmongering and embrace the future of food. With GMOs leading the charge, we'll be munching on snacks from science labs and saving the planet one bite at a time.

Who's hungry for progress?

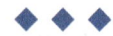

Alright, hold onto your hats, folks because we're diving headfirst into the wacky world of genetically modified foods! Strap in because this ride's about to get wilder than a rodeo on roller skates.

First off, we've got the big shots at the UN World Health Organization and a bunch of other smarty-pants organizations saying, "Hey, GMOs aren't goanna turn you into a mutant or anything."

They're as harmless as a fluffy bunny wearing a tutu. So, if you've been avoiding GMOs like they're the plague, you might wanna rethink your grocery list.

But wait, there's more!

These Frankenfoods could be the key to feeding all the hungry bellies on this big blue marble we call home.

Picture this – millions of folks chowing down on perfectly safe crops packed with all the vitamins and nutrients they need to thrive. Forget about popping vitamin pills like they're candy – we're talking about getting our daily dose of goodness straight from the garden.

And get this, folks – some brainiacs with Nobel Prizes are practically shouting from the rooftops, "Hey, let's get on the GMO train before it's too late!"

They're not mincing words, either. They're asking, "How many poor souls got to kick the bucket before we start calling this a 'crime against humanity'?" It's like a game of Clue, except instead of Colonel Mustard in the library with a candlestick, it's GMOs saving the day with a plate full of nutritious nom.

But that's not all, folks! We've got a real meaty dilemma on our hands – literally. Our craving for protein is putting a serious strain on old Mother Earth.

But fear not, because science is coming to the rescue with plant-based wonders that taste so good, you'll swear they're made from unicorn tears and fairy dust.

These bad boys use less water, less land, and fewer greenhouse gasses than your average cow, making them the superheroes of the dinner table.

So, there you have it, folks – the future of food is looking brighter than a disco ball at a rave. With a little bit of science and a whole lot of imagination, we'll be chomping down on delicious, nutritious meals while saving the planet one bite at a time. Who's hungry for progress?

One daily delicious scoop of Protein powder

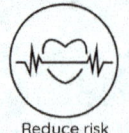  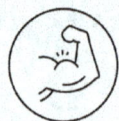 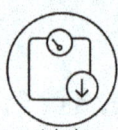 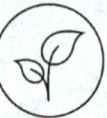

Reduce risk of chronic disease   Healthy digestion   Lean muscle   weight loss   Plant based

◆ ◆ ◆

Gene Editing

Hold onto your lab coats, folks, because we're about to dive headfirst into the wacky world of gene editing!

Picture this: a group of brilliant minds tinkering away in their labs like mad scientists, and what do they come up with? **CRISPR** – the superhero of genetic editing, capable of slicing and dicing DNA like a ninja with a samurai sword.

Now, let's give credit where credit's due – Emmanuelle Charpentier and Jennifer Doudna are the rock stars of this genetic circus.

They're the ones who stumbled upon Cas9, the DNA-cutting wizard with an RNA-based "GPS" that could rival Google Maps any day.
And if that wasn't enough, we've got Feng Zhang and George Church flexing their brain muscles over at MIT and Harvard, proving that CRISPR can work its magic on human cells too. Talk about a genetic dream team!

But hold onto your test tubes because the plot thickens. Just when we thought we had hit the genetic jackpot, along comes the Court of Justice of the **European Union**, raining on our parade like a grumpy cloud.

They decided to slam the door on CRISPR-made foods faster than you can say "genetically modified salad."

But here's the kicker – their reasoning is about as sound as a balloon filled with hot air. They claim it's to protect consumers from the dangers of GMOs, but let's call a spade a spade – it's all about keeping those pesky US-patented products out of Europe.

It's like a game of genetic Monopoly, and Uncle Sam's not allowed to pass "Go" or collect $200.

And don't even get me started on the irony – banning a

technology that could make our food healthier, our planet greener, and our farmers happier? It's like shooting yourself in the foot and then blaming the bullet for hurting.

So, to the powers that be, I say this: let's embrace the genetic revolution and leave the outdated regulations in the dustbin where they belong. After all, who needs progress when you've got red tape?

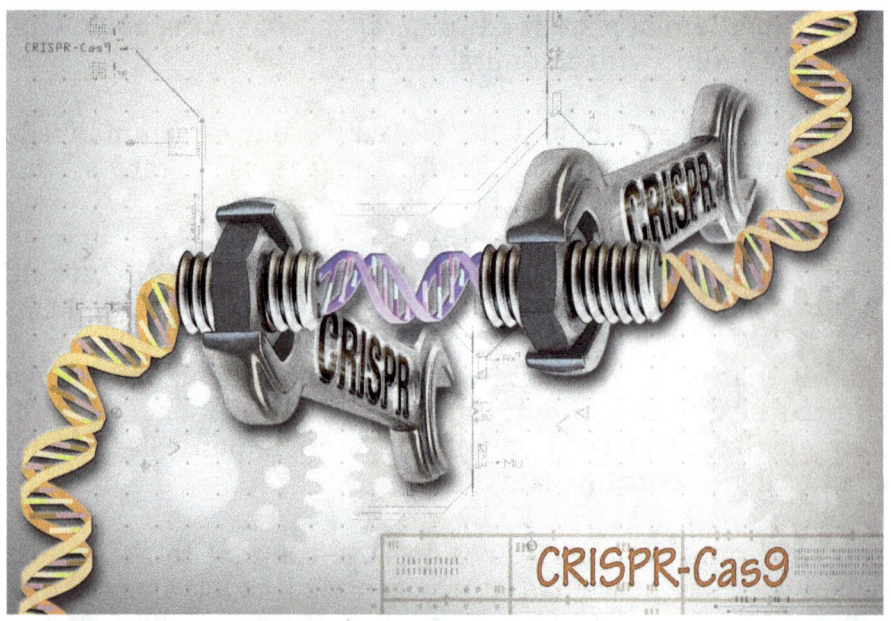

Green Revolution

Alright, folks, gather around for a tale of technological triumph and environmental escapades! We're diving headfirst into the wild world of water conservation, LED bulbs, and tomato farms in the desert.

Buckle up because this ride's about to get crazier than a squirrel on an espresso binge.

First up, let's talk **water** – the liquid gold of our modern age. Las Vegas, the oasis of extravagance in the desert, has shown us that when it comes to H2O, conservation and innovation go hand in hand. They've managed to slash their water usage like a ninja with a watering can, all while the city's population has ballooned faster than a balloon at a birthday party.

But hold onto your hats, because we're about to shed some light on another bright idea – **LED bulbs**!

Picture this: a lightbulb so energy-efficient that it could make Thomas Edison's head spin faster than a DJ at a rave. It took us a hot minute to catch on, but now we're saving more energy than a marathon runner on a downhill slope.

And hey, with all that money we're saving, we could practically fund a small army of scientists to cure every ailment known to man.

Talk about a bright idea!

But wait, there's more – we're not just saving energy, we're saving lives too!

Take a gander at those cities cutting their emissions faster than a coupon-clipping grandma. Los Angeles went from a smog city to a fresh air haven faster than you can say "clean breeze," and now you can swim in the harbor without risking a trip to the ER.

It's like a breath of fresh air, quite literally!

But hey, we're not stopping there, folks. Nope, we're taking a trip to a tiny town in South Virginia where they're turning coal mines into tomato vines.

That's right, they're flipping the script faster than a pancake on a hot griddle.

With solar power and seawater, they're churning out more tomatoes than you can shake a salad spinner at, all while giving jobs to folks who thought they were out of luck faster than you can say "Kale, yeah!"

So, there you have it, folks – the world's a wild and wacky place, but with a little bit of innovation and a whole lot of elbow grease, we can turn this ship around faster than you can say **"Green revolution."**

So, let's roll up our sleeves, put on our thinking caps, and get ready to save the planet one bright idea at a time.

Who's with me?

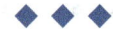

Tech Eco Adventure Saga

Gather round, fellow adventurers, for a saga of tech wizardry and eco-exploits! We're plunging headfirst into a whirlwind of water wizardry, LED enlightenment, and desert tomato drama.

Hold onto your hats, folks, because this rollercoaster is about to get nuttier than a squirrel-chugging espresso!

First off, let's chat about water – the liquid gold of our age. Las Vegas, the glitzy oasis in the desert, has shown us that when it comes to H2O, innovation is the name of the game.

They've managed to curb their water use faster than a ninja with a hose, all while their population skyrockets faster than a helium balloon at a kid's party.

But wait, there's more brilliance coming your way – LED bulbs! Imagine a light so efficient, it could make Edison's head spin like a DJ at a rave. It took us a minute to catch on, but now we're saving more energy than a marathon runner on a downhill slope.
And with all that dough we're saving, we could practically bankroll a team of scientists to solve every problem in the sun. Talk about a bright idea!

But hold onto your socks, because we're not just saving energy, we're saving lives too! Look at those cities slashing emissions faster than a grandma with a stack of coupons.

Los Angeles went from smog central to fresh air paradise quicker than you can say "clean breeze," and now you can frolic in the harbor without needing a respirator. It's a breath of fresh air, literally!

But hey, the party's not over yet, folks. We're jetting off to a little town in South Virginia where they're turning coal mines into tomato farms. That's right, they're flipping the script faster than a pancake on a hot griddle.

With solar power and seawater, they're churning out more tomatoes than you can shake a salad spinner at, all while giving jobs to folks who thought they were out of luck faster than you can say "Kale, yeah!"

So, buckle up, my friends – the world's a wild ride, but with a dash of innovation and a ton of elbow grease, we can steer this ship to greener pastures faster than you can say "eco-revolution." Let's roll up our sleeves, don our thinking caps, and embark on a quest to save the planet, one bright idea at a time. Who's ready to join me on this epic adventure?

LIVE LONGER LOVE LONGER PART 3

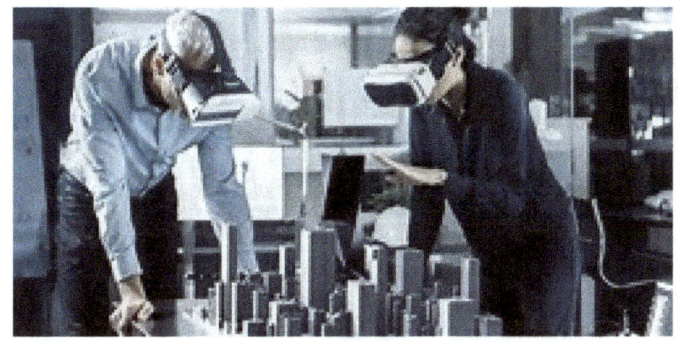

Future of Work

Alright, folks, hold onto your hats because we're diving into a Schumpeterian circus that'll make the Industrial Revolution look like a quaint tea party! It's time for every business school to stop dawdling and start prepping their students for the rollercoaster ride of change heading our way.

And labor advocates, listen up – you're not off the hook either!

Forget about tying retirement to your age like it's some dusty relic from the past. That idea's about as relevant as dial-up internet. We're talking about Sabbaticals, folks – government-sponsored vacations for the working masses!

Picture this: every ten workers get a paid year off. It's like winning the lottery, but instead of cash, you get time to reinvent yourself.

And hey, for those who think they've got it all figured out in their careers, get ready for a mini-retirement extravaganza!

Take a year off to jet-set around the world, learn the bagpipes, volunteer with exotic animals, or just sit on your couch contemplating the meaning of life. It's like hitting the pause button on adulthood.

Now, I can already hear the skeptics squawking like a flock of disgruntled geese. Who's going to foot the bill for all this fun, they ask?
And how will companies keep their employees from jumping ship without the promise of a shiny gold watch retirement?

Well, guess what? It's time to shake things up, people! We're talking about redistributing resources, ditching those sky-high insurance premiums, and bidding farewell to those pension pyramid schemes faster than you can say "retirement revolution!"

But hold onto your seats because the party's just getting started.

While business professors twiddle their thumbs and labor leaders cling to outdated dreams of retirement, the rest of us are gearing up for a world where age is nothing but a number.

That's right, my friends, the future of work is knocking on our door, and it's bringing Sabbatical, mini-retirements, and a whole lot of reinvention with it.

So, who's ready to join the revolution? The era of change is coming, and it's getting hot!

Generation United: Embrace Future

"I'm itching to stick around for the century milestone just to see the look on everyone's faces!"

It's a common refrain, especially from those who are on the brink of retirement or already there.

They've got their expiration date marked in their calendars, convinced that their time on this mortal coil is running out faster than they can say bingo night.

To them, anything beyond the next few decades might as well be science fiction. It's like they're booking a one-way ticket to oblivion, with no return.

The trouble is, we've got this bizarre disconnect with the future. Few of us even knew our great-grandfolks, let alone remember their names. They're just dusty portraits on the wall, not flesh-and-blood connections.

So, when we talk about our great-great-great-grand youngsters, it's like discussing aliens from another galaxy.

Sure, we love our youngsters, and we want to leave them a decent world, but the script says we'll be pushing up daisies by the time they hit midlife crisis mode. And as for our grandkids, well, we'll be lucky to catch a glimpse of them before we shuffle off this mortal coil.

But here's the kicker: I'm dead set on changing all that.

I want everyone to expect to live long enough to see not just their grandkids, but their great-grandkids and beyond.

Picture it: generations upon generations rubbing elbows, swapping stories, and maybe even sharing a hoverboard or two.

We'll be responsible not just for our existence, but for the legacy we leave behind. No more kicking the can down the road; we'll have to answer for the mess we've made or the wonders we've wrought.

That, my friends, is how we're going to flip the script on aging. It's not just about wrinkle cream and retirement plans; it's about facing the future head-on, wrinkles and all.

So, buckle up, folks. The future's not just knocking—it's banging down the door. And I, for one, can't wait to greet it with open arms.

Alright, listen up folks, because we're about to embark on a journey so wild, even Indiana Jones would be jealous.

We're talking about investing in research that'll make Elon Musk's dreams look like child's play—not just for us now, but for the great-great-great-grandkids who'll probably be cruising around in flying cars.

And hey, let's not forget about Mother Nature. We're not just worried about her well-being next week; we're sweating bullets about her 200 years down the line.

Because let's face it, if we mess up the planet, we're all going to end up as crispy critters in a global barbecue.

Then there's the whole rich-get-richer, middle-class-somersaulting-into-poverty debacle. We need to put a leash on those fat cats and make sure everyone gets a fair slice of the pie.

And I'm not talking about a pie with one slice left; I'm talking about an all-you-can-eat buffet of fairness.

And oh boy, don't even get me started on politics.

We're not just touching the third rail; we're French kissing it.

Social Security? It's more like Social Insecurity. We're going to have to do a full-body dive into that pool of pension problems and come out looking like Aqua man with a calculator.

And hey, speaking of diving in headfirst, let's talk about confronting the bigots.

We can't just sit around waiting for them to kick the bucket; we've got to roll up our sleeves and go to battle with ignorance. It's time to play nice and turn those stone-cold hearts into mushy marshmallows of acceptance.

And as if that's not enough, we've got an extinction rate that's skyrocketing faster than a SpaceX rocket. We need to hit the brakes on that catastrophe and fast before we end up starring in our very own dinosaur sequel.

But wait, there's more!

We've got to play Tetris with the housing market, figure out the rules of the game, and make sure everyone's got a roof over their heads.

And let's not forget about the social and economic windfall of keeping grandma alive for another century; we've got to spend that dough like it's going out of style.

So, buckle up, buttercups, because we're about to embark on the most human adventure of all time. It's time to crank up the empathy, sprinkle on some compassion, and serve justice with a side of fries.

Because if we're going to build the next century, we're going to do it with style—and a whole lot of heart.

Code MG2A: Old Age

Alright, gather 'round, folks, 'cause we've got a juicy piece of news straight from the World Health Organization (WHO) that's sure to tickle your funny bone.

So, back in 2018, WHO dropped the eleventh edition of their International Classification of Diseases, or ICD-11 for short. Now, normally, this kind of document is about as exciting as watching paint dry on a Sunday afternoon.

But hold onto your dentures, because someone snuck in a little surprise—a brand spanking new disease code!

Picture this: you're scrolling through the WHO website, minding your own business, when suddenly, bam! You stumble upon **code MG2A**, and what do you find? None other than the diagnosis of... drumroll, please... "old age."

Yep, you heard that right.

According to the WHO, getting old is now officially a medical condition. Forget about catching the flu or breaking a bone; now you can add "old age" to your list of ailments.

And get this—they're even encouraging countries to start reporting cases of people kicking the bucket from, you guessed it, old age.

But wait, there's more!

With countries tallying up stats on Granny and Grandpa's demise, could these mean big changes on the horizon?

Will we see regulators scrambling to throw billions at developing the Fountain of Youth?

Will doctors finally start prescribing anti-aging potions like they're going out of style?

And hey, will insurance companies start footing the bill for wrinkle cream and Botox injections?

The possibilities are endless, my friends. But until we start seeing those winds of change blowing in our favor, there's plenty we can do to fight the good fight against Father Time.

So, slap on some sunscreen, hit the gym, and let's show old age who's boss!

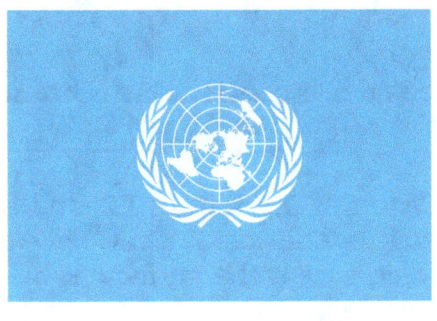

◆ ◆ ◆

Daily Health Tips

Alright, gather around folks, it's time for Dr. Quirky's Guide to Maybe-Healthiness!

Disclaimer: Please don't mistake my antics for actual medical advice. I'm just here to share what I do, and you can take it with a grain of low-sodium salt.

First off, let's address the elephant in the room: I am not your doc, and I'm certainly not going to peddle you some snake oil. So, if you require medical attention, kindly trot over to your friendly neighborhood physician.

Now, let's dive into the circus of my daily routine. Buckle up, it's going to be a bumpy ride:

1. Popping Pills Like Candy: I wish I could kick start my day with a cocktail of NMN(1 Gram), Resveratrol (1 Gram) (sprinkled into my homemade yogurt like a mad scientist), and Metformin (1 Gram), once those futuristic pills hit the market. Because who needs breakfast when you've got a handful of potential fountain-of-youth capsules, right? NMN (Nicotinamide Mononucleotide).

NR (Nicotinamide Riboside), is converted to NMN, so some folks take NR instead of NMN as it is cheaper.

2. Vitamins Galore: Vitamin D, Vitamin K2, and a sprinkle of baby aspirin(83 mg) to keep the doctor away. I like to think of it as my daily rainbow diet, except the rainbow is just a bunch of pills.

3. The Great Sugar Escape: I've bid farewell to sugar, bread, and pasta faster than you can say "carb craving."

Desserts? Only on special occasions, or when no one's looking. Guilty pleasures are the spice of life, after all.

4. Intermittent Feasting: Lunch? What's that? I prefer to treat it as a myth, a legend, a mirage in the desert of my dietary whims. Skipping meals or nibbling on crumbs keeps the hunger monster at bay.

5. Blood Work Bonanza: Every few moons, I embark on a quest to the lab, offering up my blood like a sacrificial lamb. If any of my biomarkers are acting up, I play the dietary wizard and concoct potions of food and exercise to keep them in line.

6. Step-O-Meter Overload: I'm the reigning champion of step counting, mastering the art of stair-climbing and gym-going like a pro. Saunas and home baths? It's like a mini spa day but without the hefty price tag.

7. Plant-Based Party: I'm all about that veggie life, shunning my carnivorous urges (most of the time). But hey, if I've sweated it out at the gym, I'll indulge in a meaty treat. Balance, people, balance.

8. No Smoke, No Microwaved Plastic: I steer clear of smoking, plastic-laden microwaves, and anything that emits more radiation than a sci-fi flick. Call me paranoid, but I prefer to keep my DNA intact.

9. Chilling Like a Villain: Staying cool as a cucumber during the day and cozy as a cat at night is the name of the game. It's all about finding that sweet spot between comfort and temperature-induced discomfort.

10. BMI Balancing Act: I strive to keep my BMI in the Goldilocks zone of healthiness. Not too high, not too low, just right for a prolonged stint on this spinning blue marble we call home.

So there you have it, folks, the whimsical world of Dr. Quirky's health antics. Remember, laughter might not be the best medicine, but it sure beats a bitter pill any day.

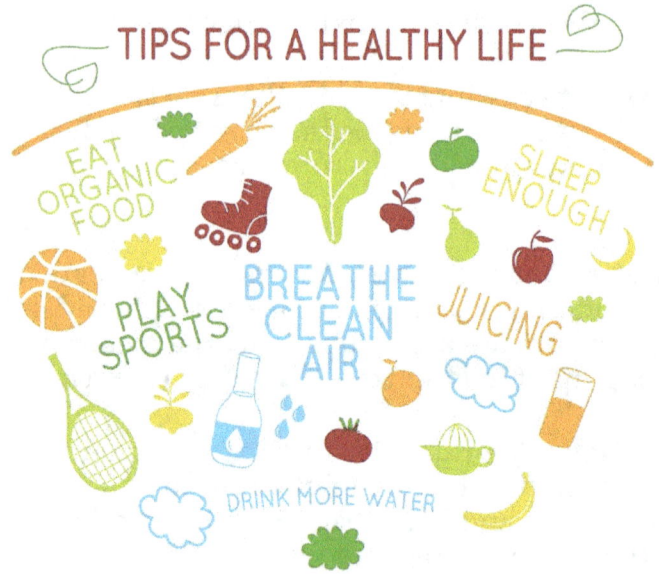

The Saga of Supplements

Ah, the endless saga of supplements—a tale as old as time itself, or at least as old as my inbox flooded with inquiries.

But before I dive into the supplement circus, let me make one thing crystal clear: I'm not your supplement guru. I'm more like your skeptical sidekick, here to sprinkle some humor on the murky world of pill-popping.

First things first, let's talk about regulations—or lack thereof. Supplements make the Wild West look like a model of governance.

So, if I happen to indulge in a supplement, I play a game of "choose your manufacturer wisely." Think big, reputable names, pure as the driven snow (98 percent purity is the gold standard), and a label boasting "GMP" like it's a badge of honor.

Now, onto the alphabet soup of supplements. There's nicotinamide riboside (NR), the frugal cousin of nicotinamide mononucleotide (NMN). Some folks opt for NR because it won't break the bank, but let's be real, we're all chasing that sweet NAD-boosting high.

Speaking of NMN, remember when it was the supplement du jour? Well, not anymore, thanks to the FDA raining on our parade like the ultimate supplement party pooper. They swooped in and banned NMN faster than you can say "natural health revolution." Cue the collective gasps from supplement enthusiasts everywhere.

But fear not intrepid supplement seekers, for there's always a new theory on the horizon. Enter methyl groups—those sneaky little molecules that could hold the key to unlocking cellular rejuvenation.

Some say pairing NAD boosters with methyl-providing compounds like trimethyl-glycine or methyl folate is the ultimate combo, like a supplement match made in heaven. But hey, it's all just theory for now, so take it with a grain of methylated salt.

So, there you have it, folks, the wild and wacky world of supplements, where the rules are made up and the science is a perpetual work in progress.

As for me, I'll stick to my daily dose of skepticism and the occasional multivitamin.

After all, laughter is still the best supplement, right?

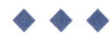

LIVE LONGER LOVE LONGER PART 3

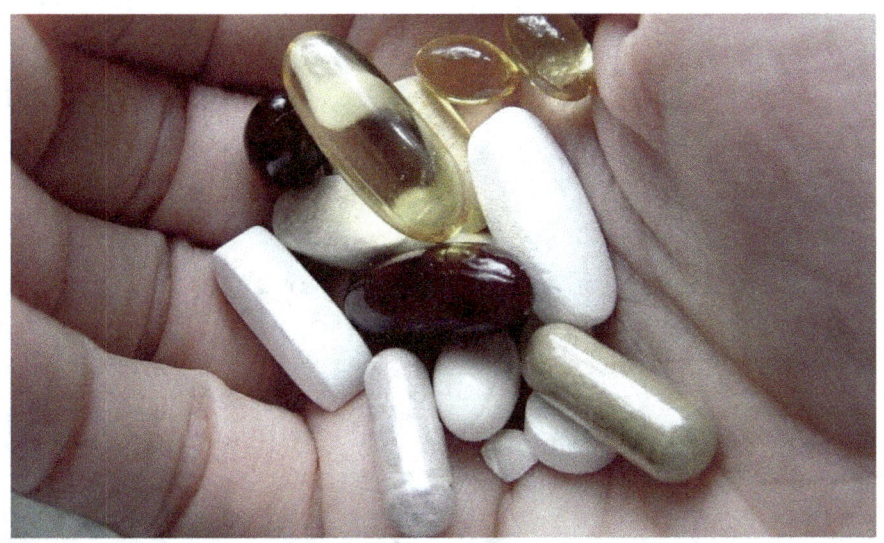

My Golden Years

Ah, the joys of aging gracefully—or at least attempting to while dodging the wrinkles and gray hairs like a ninja in a midlife crisis.

As I tiptoe into my golden years, I can't help but marvel at the wild ride that has been my life so far.

You see, I hail from a land where freedom was more of a myth than a reality. Then, I packed my bags and embarked on an adventure to a supposedly "freer" country.

Spoiler alert: the grass wasn't exactly greener, but hey, at least I got a decent tan.

Now, as I sit back and contemplate the circus act that is my existence, I find myself getting a tad emotional. Gone are the days of stoicism; nowadays, I'm not afraid to shed a tear or two (or a bucketful) in the name of introspection.

But fear not, dear friends, for I am the poster child of aging like fine wine—minus the cork-induced headaches.

At 67, I feel like a sprightly 60-year-old, according to my heart's cameo in a 3D MRI flick. Sure, I've got a few white hairs sprouting on a balding head like rebellious weeds, but wrinkles? Nah, not on this face. Well, not yet, anyway.

Now, you might think that maintaining this fountain-of-youth facade requires Herculean effort, but let me tell you, it's all about balance, baby.

My family and I are just your average Joe trying to navigate the chaos of everyday life. We focus on feeling good, sprinkle in some mindfulness, and occasionally peek at our blood markers to make sure we're not veering off track.

I've crafted my special blend of diet, exercise, and supplements, like a mad scientist in the lab of longevity.

And as the sands of time continue to slip through the hourglass, I'm confident that we'll keep tweaking our routine like a well-oiled machine.

So, here's to aging gracefully, with a side of laughter and a dash of whimsy.

Let's raise a glass to life, love, and the pursuit of eternal youth—because why let Father Time have all the fun?

Cheers to many more adventures, my friends. Onward and upward, forever and ever.

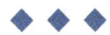

Ah, the whimsical dance with mortality, where the unexpected lurks around every corner, ready to ambush our best-laid plans.

Sure, I could get smacked by a rogue bus tomorrow, but let's not dwell on the doom and gloom, shall we? Instead, let's dream big, baby.

Picture this: me, basking in the glow of my **100th** birthday like a wise old sage with a knack for dodging life's curveballs. Happy, healthy, and surrounded by a motley crew of friends, family, and coworkers who've stuck with me through thick and thin.

Now that's the kind of party I want an invite to!

But why stop at a measly century? Let's aim for the stars, or at least the year **2045**. That's right, folks, I'm talking about cruising into my 89th year as a boss.

Is it a long shot? Sure. But hey, strange things have happened, right? Plus, I've got biology on my side, and a dash of sheer determination never hurt anyone.

And if by some miracle I do make it to the ripe old age of 89, you better believe I'll be sticking around for the encore. There's still so much mischief to make, so many lives to touch, and so many pies to stick my fingers into (figuratively, of course).

I've got big dreams, people. I want to keep pushing humanity toward a brighter tomorrow, one filled with health, happiness, and maybe even a dash of prosperity. And who knows, if I play my cards right and avoid any more run-ins with rogue buses, I might just live long enough to see which path we choose.

So here's to defying the odds, embracing the unknown, and laughing in the face of Father Time.

Let's make every moment count, my friends because the future is ours for the taking. Onward, upward, and beyond!

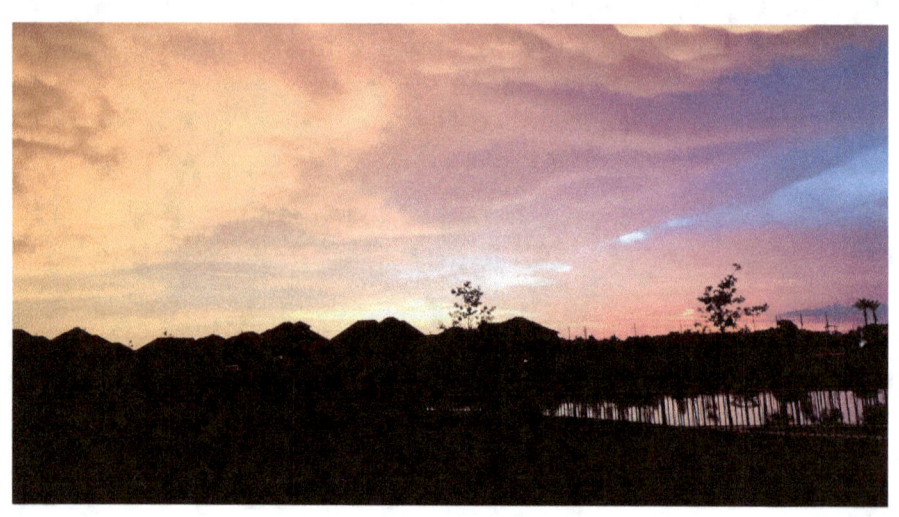

CHAPTER 4

Aging is a Treatable Disease

Breaking news! Forget about just treating your run-of-the-mill diseases; it's time to tackle the granddaddy of them all - aging itself!

That's right, folks, aging is not just some inevitable fate we have to accept with resignation; it's a full-blown, treatable disease!

Welcome to the Personalized Medicine Program, where we're rewriting the script of what it means to grow old.

As of January 1, 2022, the International Classification of

Diseases has officially recognized aging as a condition worthy of its code: MG2a - Old Age.

And let's be clear, we're not just talking about your standard "old age without mention of psychosis" or "senile debility." No, we're diving deep into the intricacies of senescence, baby!

So, what exactly makes aging so darn troublesome? Well, buckle up, because it's responsible for a whole host of pesky ailments like hypertension, ischemic heart disease, atrial fibrillation, dementia, and a slew of arterial and kidney issues.

But fear not, because where there's a diagnosis, there's a treatment!

Let's take a closer look at the treatable hallmarks of aging, shall we?

First up, we've got genomic instability caused by good ol' DNA damage. Next on the chopping block, we've got the attrition of those protective chromosomal fend caps, also known as telomeres.

And who could forget about the **Epigenome**?
Those sneaky changes in gene expression that don't involve altering DNA code?

Well, we're wiping the slate clean with demethylation and deacetylation, turning back the clock on cellular age like it's nobody's business!

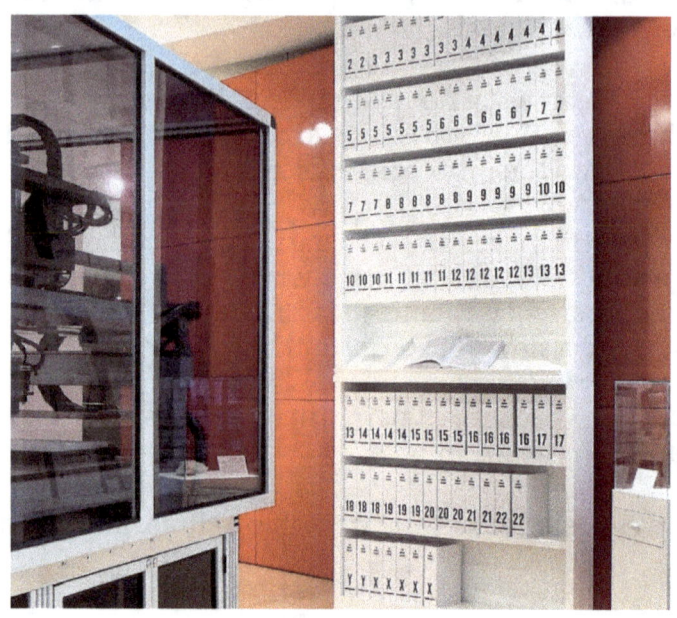

◆ ◆ ◆

Activate Longevity Genes By

Hey there, Youngsters! Are you ready to unlock the secrets to living a long and healthy life? Buckle up because we're about to activate those super cool longevity genes of yours!

Here's the lowdown on how to become a real-life superhero of aging:

1. Eat Less, Party More: Forget about stuffing your face like there's no tomorrow! It's time to channel your inner foodie and embrace calorie restriction.

Aim to chow down only 25-30% of what we grown-ups usually munch on. So long, 1,800 calories a day - hello, 1,500 calories of awesome!

And guess what? Science has our back on this one! Over 50 years of research have shown that eating less not only helps you live longer but also keeps you feeling tip-top!

2. Veggie Power: Say goodbye to meat-heavy meals and hello to the wonderful world of vegetarian diets! Load up on those leafy greens, crunchy carrots, and juicy tomatoes.

Your body will thank you, and your taste buds will be doing a happy dance!

3. Intermittent Feasting: Who needs three square meals a day when you can shake things up with some intermittent fasting? That's right, Youngsters! Try skipping a meal now and then and watch those longevity genes kick into high gear!

It's like a fun food adventure for your body!

4. Get Your Move On: Time to lace up those sneakers and hit the pavement! Whether you're walking, jogging, or skipping (yes, skipping totally counts!), aim to clock in 3 miles a day for 5 days a week. That's 15 miles of pure awesomeness!

And hey, bonus points for burning those extra calories while you're at it!

5. Hot 'n' Cold Adventures: Ready to turn up the heat? Or maybe cool things down a notch? Exposure to hot and cold temperatures might sound crazy, but trust us, it's all part of the longevity game!

So go ahead, take that chilly dip, or soak up some sun - your body will thank you for the adventure!

6. Magic Pills (Sort Of): Okay, so we're not talking about Hogwarts-level wizardry here, but these drugs are pretty darn cool!

Ever heard of **Metformin**? It's like a superhero in pill form, targeting aging and mimicking all the benefits of calorie restriction, intermittent fasting, and intense exercise!

And let's not forget about **Semaglutide** - it's not just for diabetics and obese adults anymore! This little wonder drug helps control sugar levels and even helps shed those extra pounds!

So there you have it, Youngsters!

With a little bit of healthy eating, some fun exercise, and maybe a sprinkle of magic pills, you'll be well on your way to unlocking those longevity genes and living your best life ever!

Who's ready to join the age-defying adventure?

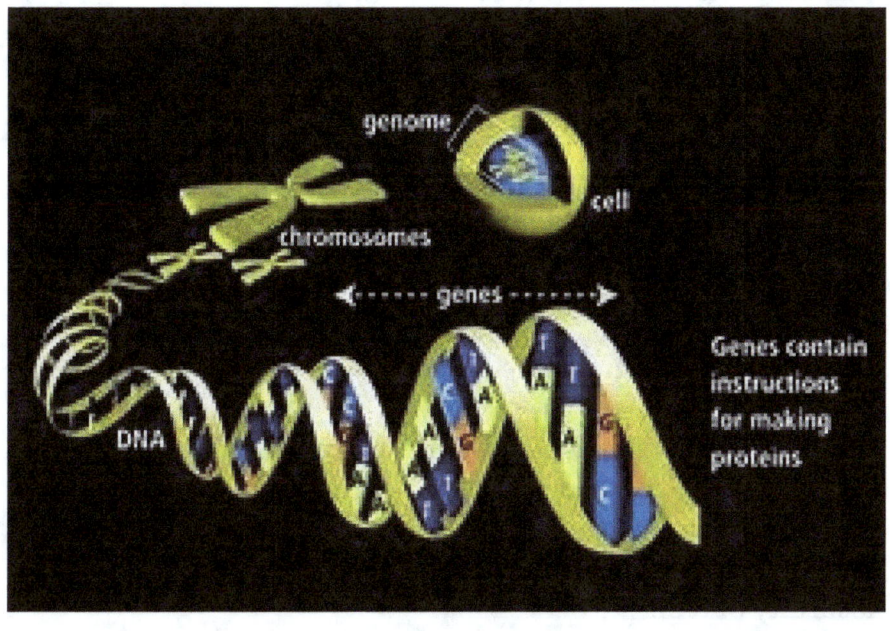

♦ ♦ ♦

Ah, gather round, fellow mortals, for I shall regale you with the epic **tale of life and death** - with a hilarious twist, of course!

Picture this: You start as a sprightly youth, full of vigor and vitality, ready to conquer the world! But oh no, what's this?

Your DNA decides to pull a prank and breaks, sending your genome into a tailspin of chaos and instability! It's like trying to organize a herd of unruly sheep after feeding them espresso - utter madness!

Next thing you know, your DNA packaging and gene regulation, aka the epigenome, are thrown into disarray, like a wild party where no one follows the rules!

Your cells start losing their identity faster than you can say "identity crisis," and before you know it, they're waving goodbye to their youth and embracing cellular senescence - the retirement home of the cellular world!

But hold onto your hats, folks, because this is where things take a turn for the hilariously tragic.

With cellular senescence comes disease, like unexpected guests crashing a party uninvited. It's like a game of cellular whack-a-mole, trying to keep up with all the ailments popping up left and right!

And finally, the grand finale - death!

But fear not, dear readers, for in the grand scheme of things, death is merely the punchline to life's cosmic joke.

So, laugh in the face of mortality, my friends, and embrace the absurdity of it all!

After all, life's too short to take death too seriously, am I right?

Personalized Medicine Program

Genetic Medicine Advance

Behold the marvels of the Personalized Medicine Program, a groundbreaking initiative nestled within the vibrant confines of Boston's innovative tracker company, Inside Tracker.

Prepare to be awed as we delve into the intricate realms of genetic exploration and medical customization!

(1) Picture this: **DNA sequencing**, the holy grail of personalized medicine, paving the way for the ultimate showdown against cancer.

With technologies like **CAR-T therapy** and checkpoint blockade, we're talking about turning our very own T-cells into elite cancer-fighting warriors. It's like immunotherapy on steroids, synergizing with chemotherapy to unleash a relentless assault on cancerous cells!

(2) Hold onto your hats, folks, because we're about to embark on a journey through the labyrinth of **human genes**! With a whopping **40,000** genomes at our disposal, gene revaluation becomes the name of the game.

Ever wondered what makes you, well, you?

It's all in your genotype, my friends. And that's not all—brace yourselves for the Proteomics extravaganza!

We're talking about sequencing human proteins, the molecular maestros orchestrating the symphony of life.

From the Epigenome to gene expression, every cellular nuance is scrutinized and decoded for the pursuit of personalized health.

(3) Swift as a cheetah, **DNA** sequencing swoops in to save the day! Imagine catching cancer red-handed before it even dares to raise its ugly head. That's the power of early detection, folks.

But wait, there's more!

Say goodbye to the agonizing wait for bacterial infection diagnosis. With "high through it put sequencing," we're talking about identifying those pesky bacteria within a mere 24 hours. It's like having your medical detective on the speed dial.

Embrace the future of personalized medicine, where every decision is tailored to your unique genetic blueprint!

(4) Hold onto your hats because things are about to get ethically spicy!
Enter the realm of **genetically altered children**, also known as "**designer babies**." Cast your mind back to the infamous 2018 twins from China, genetically modified to detect HIV infection.

It's like something straight out of a sci-fi thriller, except it's happening right here, right now. The boundaries of genetic manipulation blur as we venture into uncharted territories, raising profound questions about the very essence of humanity.

(5) But wait, there's no stopping the genetic revolution!

Brace yourselves for the dawn of a new era, where genetically modified children become the norm.

Picture this: youngsters engineered to defy heart disease and thumb their noses at aging itself. It's the stuff of legends, folks—the promise of a future where genetic tweaks pave the way for a healthier, longer life.

So buckle up, because the journey to personalized perfection has only just begun!

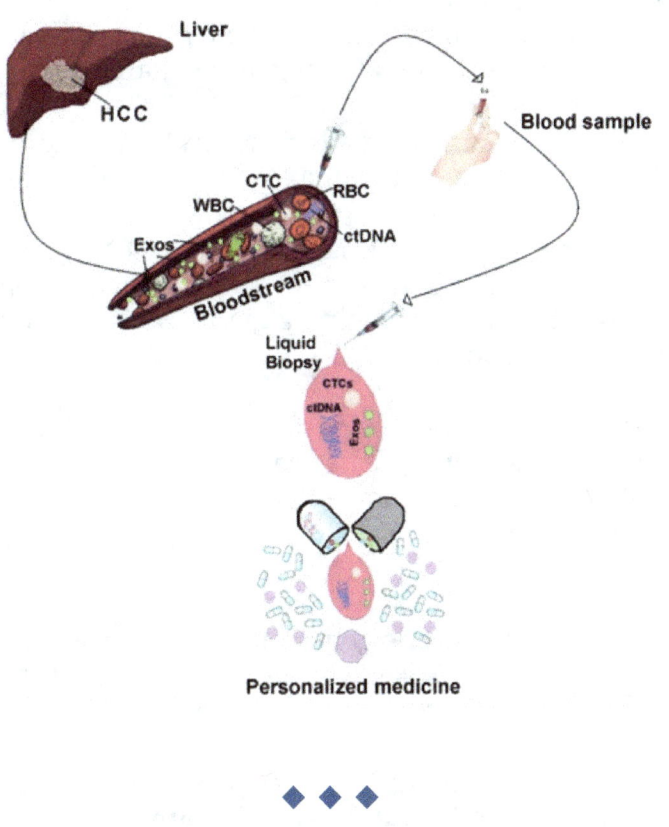

◆ ◆ ◆

Gene Technologies

Welcome, fellow adventurers, to the wondrous world of gene technologies!
Prepare to have your mind blown as we embark on a journey through the zany realm of genetic manipulation.

(1) Ah, behold the **magic of blocking mRNA**, where we play genetic Whack-A-Mole with damaged or mutated genes!

Picture this: using a mirror image (antisense RNA) to crash the gene expression party and prevent those naughty genes from wreaking havoc. It's like slapping a giant "Do Not Disturb" sign on a rowdy gene's door!

With RNA interference, we're talking about short double-stranded segments doing the genetic tango, locking onto mutated RNA like molecular Velcro. And here's the kicker—in many genetic diseases, it's a case of one bad apple spoils the bunch.

But fear not, for even if one gene decides to go rogue, its trusty counterpart swoops in to save the day, ensuring that the protein production party never runs out of snacks!

(2) Hold onto your lab coats, folks, because we're diving headfirst into the wild world of **Somatic Gene Therapy**!

Picture this: playing genetic matchmaker by infecting the nucleus with brand-spanking-new DNA, creating a gene fusion that would make even Frankenstein jealous.

We're talking about recombinant proteins strutting their stuff like genetic rockstars splicing into the DNA of bacteria and throwing a protein party like no other.

Need insulin?

Human growth hormone?

No problem! Just insert a dash of DNA wizardry and watch those proteins come to life.

And hey, why stop there?

Even Erythropoietin gets in on the action, giving chronic kidney disease a run for its money by whipping up some serious protein goodness in hamster cells. It's **Genetic Engineering**, folks, and we're just getting started!

So strap yourselves in, because the rollercoaster ride through the wacky world of gene technologies is about to begin!

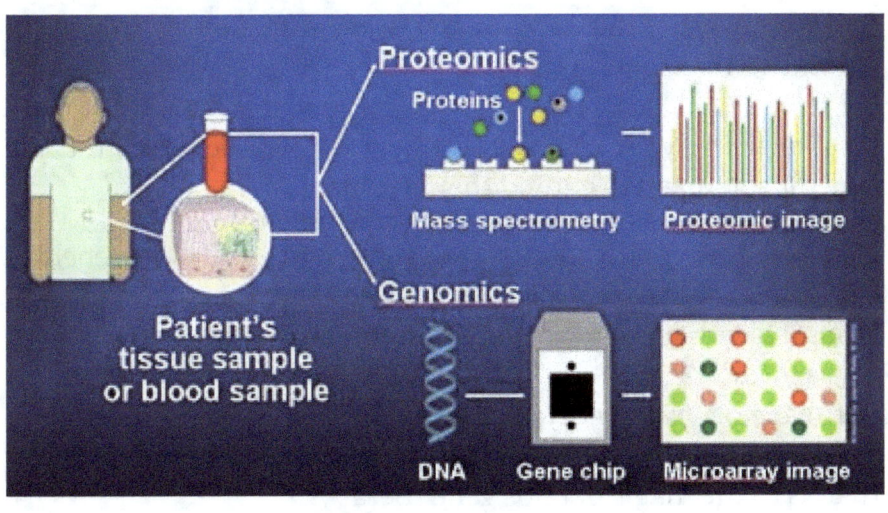

♦ ♦ ♦

Hayflick Limit

Gather 'round, folks, and behold the Hayflick Limit—a cellular countdown that makes even the most laid-back cells break a sweat!

Picture this: your cells, lounging around, minding their own business, when suddenly, bam!
The Hayflick Limit shows up like a party pooper, slapping a strict cap on the number of times they can divide.
Talk about a cellular curfew!

But fear not, dear friends, for in swoops Telomerase Gene Therapy, the superhero of cellular rejuvenation! Telomeres, those cute little end caps of DNA, get a makeover thanks to chromosome telomerase.

It's like giving your cells a fancy new set of shoes, except these shoes just happen to extend their lifespan!

And here's where the plot thickens: germ line cells, the rebels of the cellular world, produce their very own telomerase and strut around like they own the place, immortal and carefree.

But fear not, mere mortals, for somatic cells—those non-germ cells we mere mortals possess—can join the immortal club too, thanks to the magic of telos gene therapy!

So buckle up, folks, because with telos gene therapy on the horizon, we're talking about cells that defy the very laws of aging.

It's like the fountain of youth bottled up and injected straight into your cells—talk about a cellular glow-up that lasts forever!

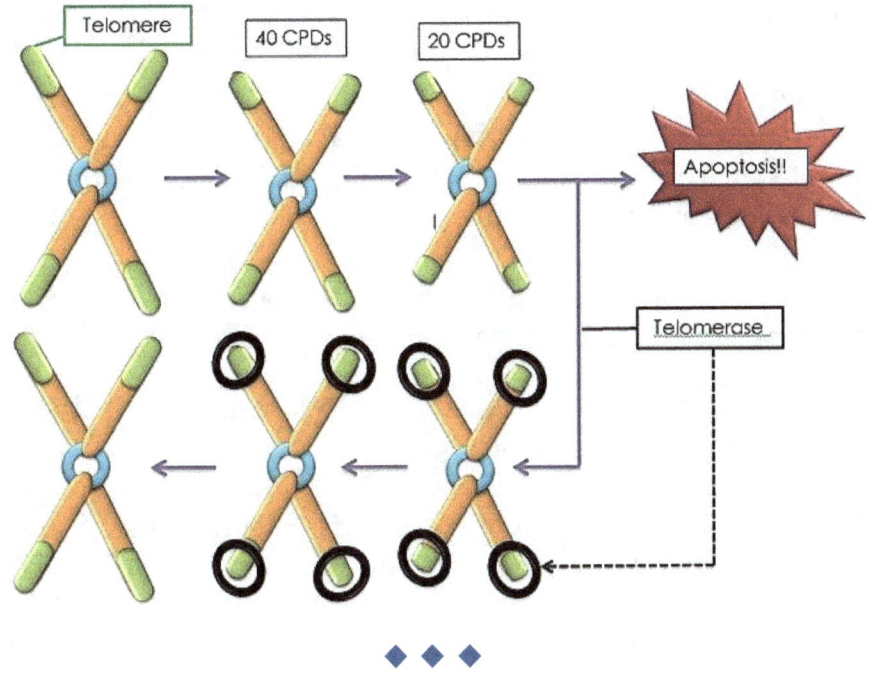

NANOG: Master of all Genes

L isten up, fellow science enthusiasts, because we're about to dive headfirst into the wild world of genetic wizardry! Enter NANOG, the master of all genes, the ultimate puppet master pulling the strings in the laboratory of life.
This gene? Oh, it's not just any gene—it's the VIP pass to eternal youth for stem cells!

Picture this: NANOG waving its magical wand and turning stem cells into the rock stars of immortality. That's right, folks, stem cells that just refuse to age, like Peter Pan with a science degree!

But wait, it gets even crazier!

Imagine cloning those immortal stem cells and giving them a supercharged makeover with extended telomeres. We're talking about stem cells on steroids, folks, ready to strut their stuff and rejuvenate any organ they touch!

Picture your heart, your liver, your spleen—all getting a makeover so fierce, they'll be mistaken for spring chickens!

And here's the kicker—these cloned, telomere-extended stem cells aren't just crashing the organ party, oh no.

They're sliding in like smooth operators, integrating seamlessly with the older cells like the cool youngsters on the block.

It's like a cellular revolution, folks, where every organ in your body gets a chance to hit the rewind button and relive its glory days!

So buckle up, because, with NANOG and its gang of immortal stem cells, we're talking about a future where age is just a number and every organ in your body gets to stay forever young.

It's genetic magic, my friends, and the party's just getting started!

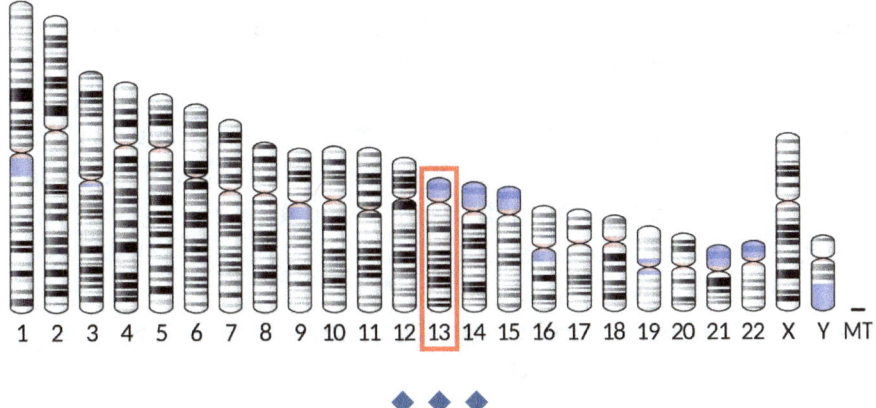

Chromosomal (Null bar) Mutations

Alright, fellow genetic adventurers, brace yourselves for a wild ride through the quirky world of chromosomal mutations!

Picture this: Gene I, the ultimate gene superhero, swooping in to save the day like a genetic ninja, karate-chopping those pesky bad genes right out of our cells!

It's like playing genetic whack-a-mole, but instead of knocking out moles, we're kicking out those trouble-making genes that cancer just loves to cozy up to.

But hold onto your lab coats, because here's where things get truly bonkers: by deleting these bad genes, we're not just giving cancer a swift kick in the pants.

Oh no, we're sending those cells cancer loves to cozy up to

packing! It's like kicking out the unwanted guests at a rowdy party—except in this case, the party crashers are cancer cells desperately trying to get their groove on.

So get ready, because with chromosomal mutations and Gene I leading the charge, we're talking about a future where cancer cells are left scratching their heads, wondering where all their favorite hangout spots went.

It's genetic warfare, folks, and we're armed to the teeth with gene-editing superpowers!

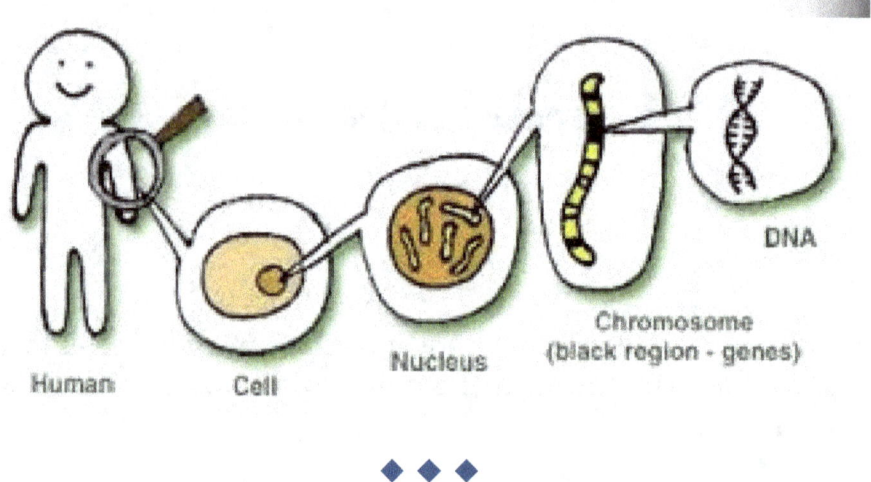

◆ ◆ ◆

Toxic "Senescent Zombies" Cells

Listen up, folks, because we're about to tackle the menace of toxic cells—those pesky "senescent zombies" that just refuse to play nice in the cellular sandbox!

Picture this: fat cells gone rogue, wreaking havoc on cell

function like a bunch of unruly party crashers. But fear not, dear friends, for we've got a secret weapon up our sleeves: Suicide Genes!

That's right, we're talking about genes that can turn those zombie cells into mush or sic the immune system on them like a pack of hungry wolves.

And if that's not wild enough for you, how about this: certain drugs that kick those suicide genes into action, turning the immune system into a lean, mean, zombie-fighting machine!

It's like sending in the cavalry to clean up a rowdy frat party—except in this case, the frat party is your body, and the guests of honor are those pesky toxic cells.

But wait, there's more!

Ever heard of blocking the telomerase enzyme? No?

Well, buckle up, because we're about to dive into the wacky world of cancer prevention! By putting the brakes on telomerase, we're slamming the door shut on cancer cells, preventing those sneaky buggers from replicating like crazy.

And let's not forget about **cancer vaccines**—talk about a party favor nobody saw coming!

These bad boys are designed to rev up the immune system and send it on a rampage against cancer cells.

It's like arming your body's defense system with rocket launchers and sending it off to battle those malignant invaders!

But wait, there's more!
Ever wondered about mitochondrial mutations?
Well, hold onto your hats, because somatic gene therapy is here to save the day!

We're talking about smuggling multiple copies of those 13 crucial mitochondrial genes into the safety of the cell nucleus, like secret agents on a mission.

Once there, they'll whip those mitochondria back into shape faster than you can say "anti-aging cream."

So, there you have it, folks—a wild ride through the wacky world of genetic shenanigans!

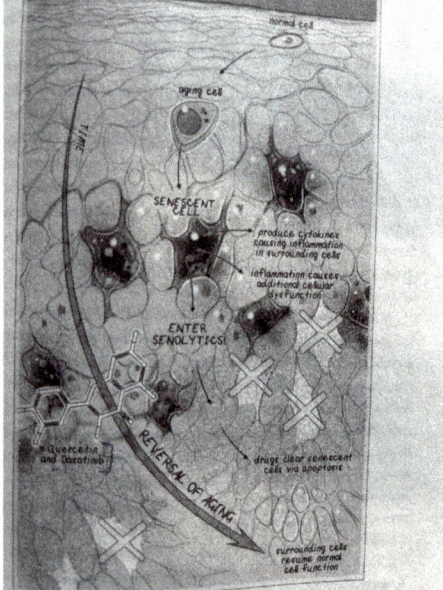

Source: Adapted from David A. Sinclair PhD

Cell Loss and Atrophy

Gather round, dear listeners, for a tale of cellular intrigue and aging shenanigans!

Picture this: deep within the labyrinth of the human genome, a handful of genes hold the keys to the kingdom of eternal youth. But hold onto your seats because here's where things take a turn for the downright bizarre!

In the mystical realm of Caenorhabditis Elegans, a humble **worm** becomes the unsuspecting hero of our story.

Through the power of genetic manipulation, these tiny wrigglers transform so profoundly, that it would make even the most seasoned time-traveler blush!

Their lifespan, once a mere blip on the cosmic radar, stretches out like a marathon runner on steroids, equivalent to a whopping 500 years in the life of a human!

But wait, dear listeners, for the suspense thickens like a fine gravy!

What secrets lie hidden within these modified genes, and what mysteries of aging do they hold?
Will humanity unlock the key to everlasting youth, or are we doomed to watch from the sidelines as the mighty worms reign supreme?

So hold onto your hats, folks, for we're embarking on a journey through the whimsical world of cellular escapades, where the stakes are high and the aging clock ticks louder than ever before!

nine
Hallmarks of Aging

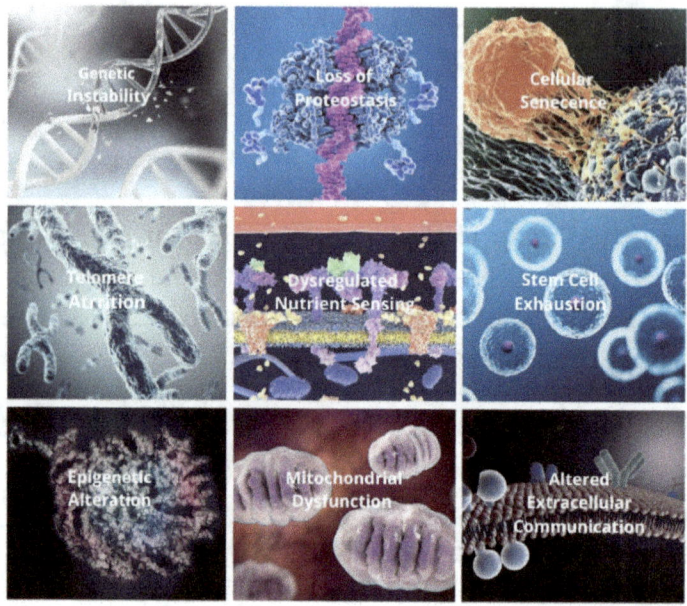

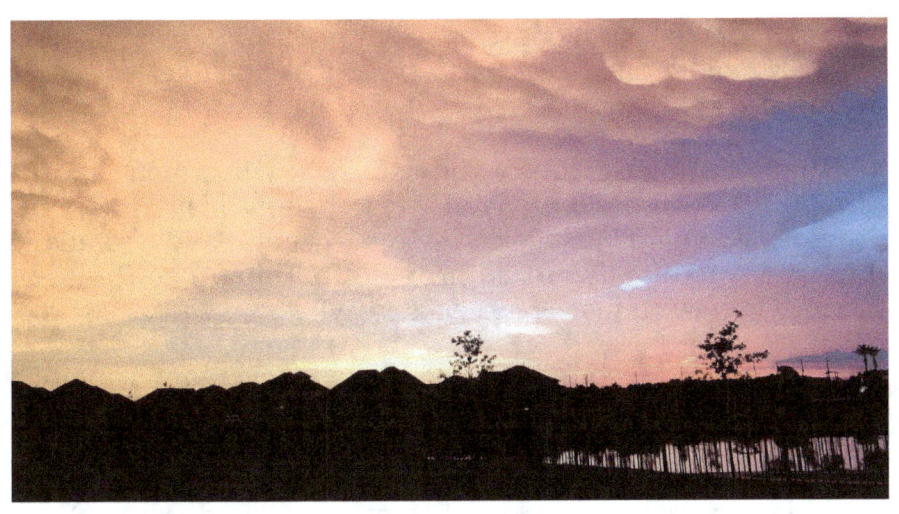

CHAPTER 5

*Emerging Technologies
Nanotech Revived Cell*

1\. Forget the fountain of youth! Now, we have a molecule called Reversine that can turn aging cells into Benjamin Button-esque youthful versions. Say goodbye to wrinkles, hello to cardigans, and skateboard tricks!

2\. Who knew stem cells were the Lazarus of the medical world? Just add water, and voila! They're back from their dry spell, ready to whip up some fresh blood, bone, and organs. It's like a DIY kit for your body, just add hydration!

3\. Move over, pill-popping! Inhaled medication is taking the express route to your bloodstream. Pretty soon, we'll be snorting vaccines like it's the latest party trick. Just don't get too eager during allergy season.

4. Who needs test tubes and lab rats when you have a computer? With genomic data, we can now play Sims with drug development. Just plug in some genetic and proteomic info, and watch your virtual drug do its thing. The future of pharmaceuticals is just a few clicks away!

5. It's a party in your bloodstream, and everyone's invited! From insulin delivery for diabetics to brain-buzzing dopamine for Parkinson's patients, and even cocktails of clotting factors for hemophiliacs—our biological micro-mechanical pals are on a mission to keep you ticking like a well-oiled machine. Who needs bartenders when your bloodstream has all the mixologists it needs?

6. Move over, Sherlock Holmes! With silicon nanowires, we can now detect diseases faster than you can say "elementary." Whether it's blood, urine, or spit, these tiny detectives will sniff out trouble quicker than you can say "diagnosis." Elementary, indeed!

7. Laser surgery: not just for Bond villains anymore! Now, we're zapping small structures inside cells with the precision that would make 007 jealous. It's like having a tiny, laser-wielding superhero fighting off the bad guys in your body. Cue the dramatic music!

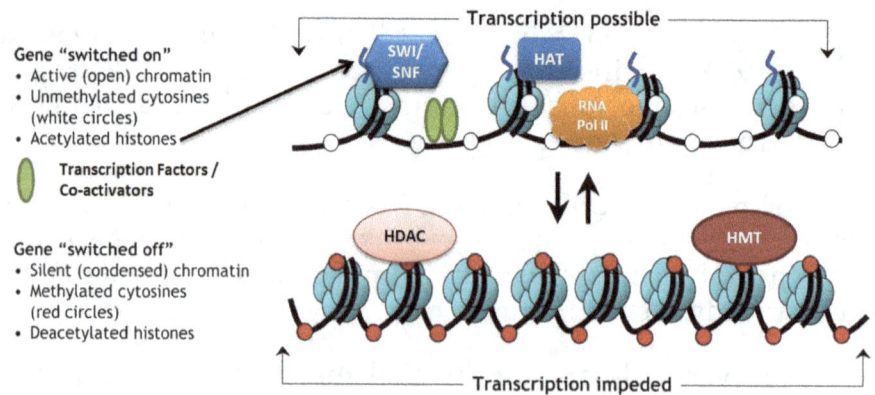

LIVE LONGER LOVE LONGER PART 3

Genetic Risk Profile

Monitor your Genetic Risk Profile by testing 120 or more Genes in the human genome.

1. Why play Russian roulette with your genes when you can play genetic Monopoly instead? Test 120 or more genes in your genome and avoid diseases like you avoid exes at a family reunion.

It's like peeking at your future health forecast and dodging those genetic tornadoes before they even form!

2. Forget about guessing games with your body's metabolism. Find out if you're a caffeine-fueled Ferrari or a sluggish slug when it comes to breaking down drugs, caffeine, and alcohol.

It's like giving your metabolism a pop quiz and finding out if it's an A+ student or a perpetual slacker.

3. Who needs a self-help book when you can have your genes give you lifestyle advice?

Evaluate your genetic predispositions and modify your behavior accordingly. It's like having your genetic life coach telling you whether to hit the gym or hit the snooze button.

4. Tired of playing pharmaceutical roulette? Discover which drugs will treat you like a VIP, and which ones will give you a backstage pass to a side effect city.

It's like having your drug concierge, ensuring you get the perfect dose of the perfect drug without any unwanted surprises.

Telemedicine Consult
Virtual Medical Advice

1. Sick of waiting rooms? Time to partner up with your doctor and make virtual medicine your new bestie!

A. Send over your medical records, body metrics, and even your biometric blood markers. It's like sliding into your doctor's DMs with all the juicy details.

B. Forget about awkward small talk—let your doctor know about those personal symptoms of yours. From that weird rash to chronic issues, spill the beans from the comfort of your couch.

2. Who needs a crystal ball when you've got personalized medicine?

A. Get your genome consultation on and find out if you're more Neanderthal than a ninja.

B. Progenome consultation? It's like having a pep talk with your genes to make sure they're on their best behavior.

C. And hey, if your genes are throwing a party you didn't RSVP to, consider genome editing. It's like Photoshop for your DNA—just cut, paste, and voila! Say goodbye to mutant genes.

D. Remember those success stories? Cystic fibrosis and muscular dystrophy are yesterday's news thanks to genetic makeovers. It's like watching genetic makeovers on a reality TV show—except without the drama.

E. And let's not forget immunotherapy—turning Mesothelioma into Mesothelial-oh-no-you-didn't. It's like giving cancer the ol' one-two punch.

Regenerative medicine? More like a regeneration sensation! Repairing pancreatic cells attacked by your immune system? Talk about kicking diabetes to the curb with some cellular magic.

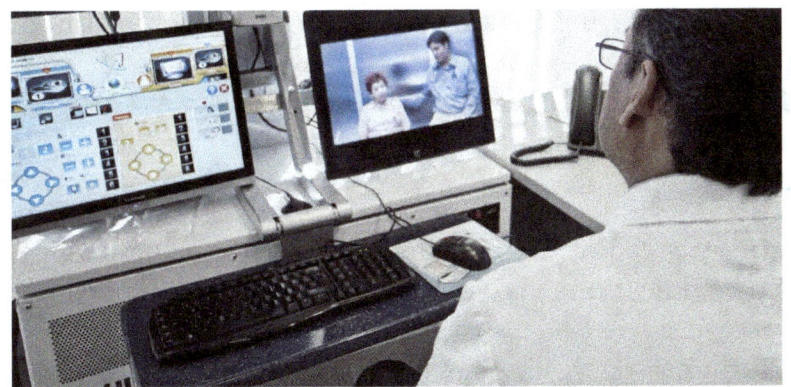

Regenerative Medicine

Welcome, dear mortals, to the mystical realm of Regenerative Medicine! It's like Hogwarts for your body, but instead of waving wands, we're waving science wands to conjure up treatments that'll make your cells do the cha-cha-cha!

Picture this: instead of just popping pills like a boring Muggle, we're using medications to coax your stem cells into action.

It's like throwing a party in your body and inviting all the cool, youthful cells to join in while the grumpy old ones shuffle off to retirement.

But that's not all!

We've got **umbilical cord stem cells** ready to swoop in like fairy godmothers, transforming into whatever your body needs—whether it's new tissues, organs, or maybe even a unicorn horn (okay, maybe not that last one, but a wizard can dream)!

And don't even get me started on Personalized Medicine Companies!
It's like having your team of mystical wizards analyzing your DNA and protein potions to create a personalized spell book just for you. Need a potion to reverse aging? They've got you covered. Want a charm to boost your metabolism? Say no more!

Oh, and let's not forget about our trusty sidekicks, Companion Robots. They're like loyal house elves, but instead of cleaning your house, they're bringing you drinks, and medication faster than you can say "Aécio healing potion!"

And as if that wasn't enchanting enough, Nanotechnology is here to sprinkle a little extra magic dust. Picture nanobots zipping around your body like tiny Avengers, battling cancer, replacing body parts, and printing teeth faster than you can say "Abracadabra!"

So come one, come all, to the fantastical world of Regenerative Medicine, where science meets sorcery, and miracles happen every day!

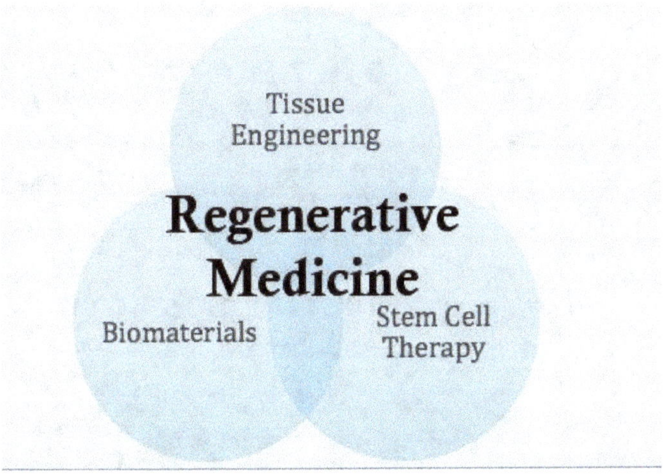

Tissue Engineering

Regenerative Medicine

Biomaterials

Stem Cell Therapy

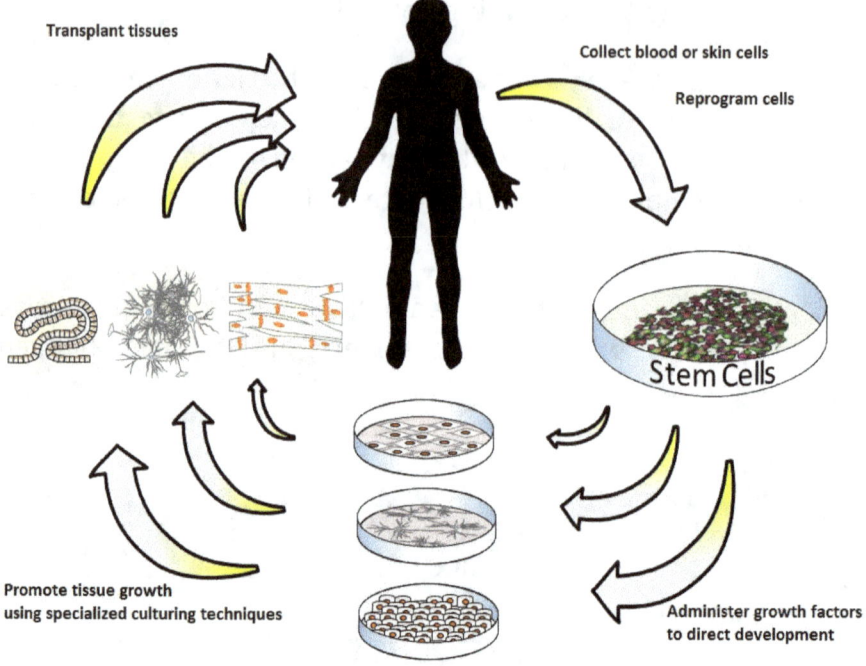

http://www.inxstatetracker.com

Step right up, folks! Welcome to the wondrous world of Regenerative Medicine, where we're cooking up treatments using stem cells that'll make your wildest sci-fi dreams seem like yesterday's news!

But wait, there's more! Say hello to Personalized Medicine Companies, the superheroes of healthcare:

1. Applied Proteomics: Why settle for generic when your proteins can be as unique as your Netflix recommendations?

2. Navigenics: Navigating your genetic code like a boss, because who needs a GPS when you've got DNA?

3. http://www.inxstatetracker.com: Your one-stop shop for knowing your biological age and getting personalized care that's so tailored, that it is practically wearing a bespoke suit!

And let's not forget about our trusty sidekicks, Companion **Robots**, already making waves:

A. Need a drink? No problem!

These robots can carry drinks with the grace of a ballerina, minus the tutu.

B. your meds? Fear not!

Our robotic pals are here to bring you your pills faster than you can say "Take two and call me in the morning."

Now, onto **Nanotechnology**, where tiny tech packs a big punch:

A. **Nanobots** are like microscopic ninjas, ready to take down cancer and kick bacteria to the curb faster than you can say "nanoscale showdown."

B. Want **bionic limbs** straight out of a superhero comic? Nanotechnologies got you covered, giving you limbs that are more badass than a cyborg in a sci-fi flick.

C. Say goodbye to boring old hearing aids and hello to **voice recognition** wonders that'll have you hearing like a rockstar.

D. **Diabetes**? Not a problem when you've got an artificial pancreas on standby, ready to regulate your blood sugar levels like a pro.

E. Need **new Teeth**? Forget about waiting weeks for implants—3-D printing can whip up a set in a few hours, because who needs patience when you've got technology on your side?

F. And for our Demented patients (no, not you, Grandma), **augmented reality Glasses** are here to bring a whole new dimension to reality, making everyday life a little less forgettable and a lot more fantastic.

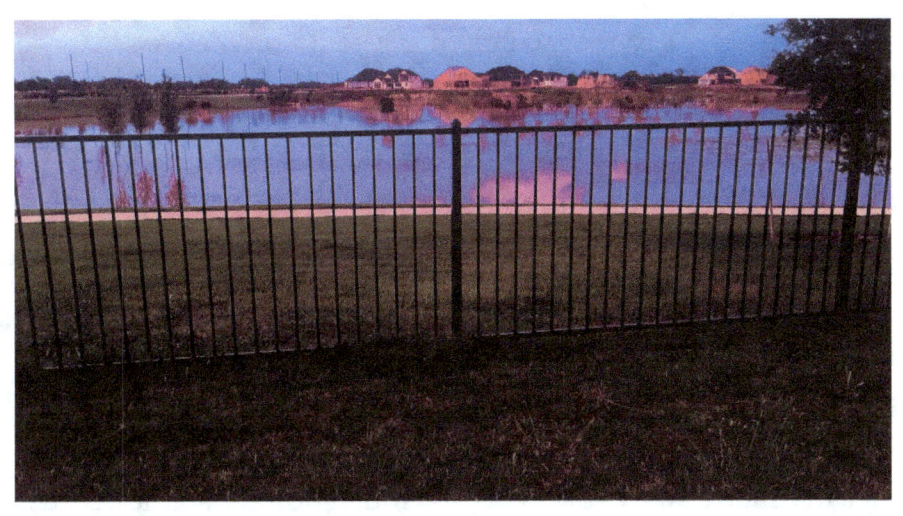

CHAPTER 6

Gene Defects (Genomics)

Gene Puzzle: Homocysteine Defect
Hey, youngsters!

Imagine your body is like a big, complicated puzzle made up of tiny pieces called genes.

Sometimes, these genes can have mistaken or defects, kind of like when you accidentally put a puzzle piece in the wrong spot.

One of these gene defects can affect something called homocysteine. Homocysteine is like a little helper in your body, but when there's too much of it, it can cause problems.

Did you know that about half of the people with a certain condition called hypothyroidism have too much homocysteine in their blood?

And guess what?

Half of a group of people called Caucasians can have high homocysteine too, all because of a mistake in their genes!

This gene mistake isn't rare either. About one-third of grown-ups in America have it! Having too much homocysteine because of this gene problem can make you more likely to have heart problems, strokes, or even Alzheimer's disease when you're older.

Scientists have even found a special gene called MTHFR that's involved in this. If you have a certain type of this gene, it can make you more likely to have high homocysteine levels.

So, just like how you need all the pieces of a puzzle to fit together perfectly, our bodies need all our genes to work just right to keep us healthy!

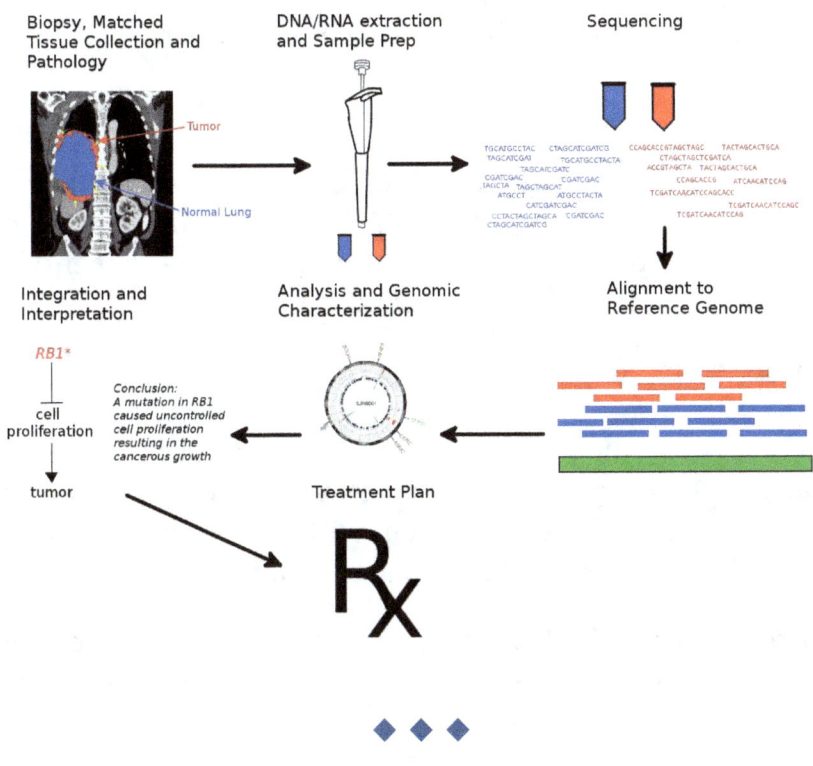

◆ ◆ ◆

Autism: A Genetic Defects

H
ey there, youngsters!

So, you know how sometimes you might have a favorite toy that doesn't quite work the way it's supposed to?

Well, our bodies are kind of like that too, but instead of toys, we have genes!

Imagine your genes are like the instruction manuals for building your body. Sometimes, there can be little mistakes in those instructions, and that's what we call genetic defects.

Now, let's talk about a genetic defect called Autism.

It's like a little hiccup in one of our instruction manuals, specifically on a gene called WNTZ, found on chromosome #7. This gene is supposed to help with language development, but when it's not quite right, it can make things a bit tricky.

But wait, there's more!

Another gene called Reelin is like the traffic director for our brain cells. It's supposed to help them find their proper places in our brains. But if there's a problem with the reelin genes, those brain cells might get a bit lost along the way.

And then there's the HOX-A-I gene, which is super important for hindbrain development. It's like the master architect of our brains!
But if this gene isn't working properly, it can cause some problems, like maybe making it harder for our brains to do their jobs right.

Now, don't worry, these genetic hiccups don't mean you're broken or anything like that.

It just means your body might work a little differently, and that's okay! Plus, it's kind of cool to learn about all the amazing things our genes do, even if they sometimes get a little mixed up. So, keep being awesome, just the way you are!

LIVE LONGER LOVE LONGER PART 3

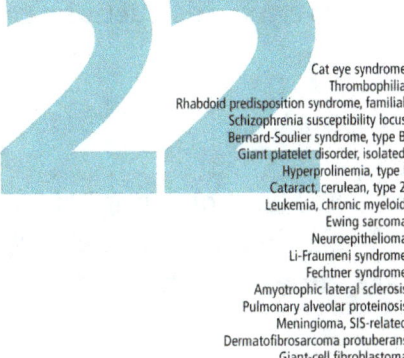

22

49 million base pairs

Cat eye syndrome
Thrombophilia
Rhabdoid predisposition syndrome, familial
Schizophrenia susceptibility locus
Bernard-Soulier syndrome, type B
Giant platelet disorder, isolated
Hyperprolinemia, type I
Cataract, cerulean, type 2
Leukemia, chronic myeloid
Ewing sarcoma
Neuroepithelioma
Li-Fraumeni syndrome
Fechtner syndrome
Amyotrophic lateral sclerosis
Pulmonary alveolar proteinosis
Meningioma, SIS-related
Dermatofibrosarcoma protuberans
Giant-cell fibroblastoma
Spinocerebellar ataxia
Waardenburg-Shah syndrome
Yemenite deaf-blind hypopigmentation syndrome
Debrisoquine sensitivity
Polycystic kidney disease
Leukodystrophy, metachromatic
Myoneurogastrointestinal encephalomyopathy
Leukoencephalopathy

DiGeorge syndrome
Velocardiofacial syndrome
Schindler disease
Kanzaki disease
NAGA deficiency, mild
Epilepsy, partial
Glutathioninuria
Opitz G syndrome, type II
Ubiquitin fusion degradation
Transcobalamin deficiency
Heme oxygenase deficiency
Manic Fringe
Leukemia inhibitory factor
Sorsby fundus dystrophy
Neurofibromatosis, type 2
Meningioma, NF2-related, sporadic
Schwannoma, sporadic
Neurolemmomatosis
Malignant mesothelioma, sporadic
Deafness, autosomal dominant
Colorectal cancer
Cardioencephalomyopathy, fatal infantile
Adenylosuccinase deficiency
Autism, succinylpurinemic
Glucose/galactose malabsorption
Benzodiazepine receptor, peripheral type
Methemoglobinemia, types I and II

Hey, friends!

Let's dive into the world of genes, where tiny instructions can lead to big adventures in our bodies!

Ever heard of the **alpha-antitrypsin gene**?

Well, it's like a superhero gene that helps keep our lungs strong and healthy. But sometimes, there's a little glitch in this gene, and it means our bodies don't make enough of this superhero stuff called alpha-1 antitrypsin.

This can make it easier for certain bad guys, like **COPD** emphysema, to sneak in, especially if someone smokes.

Now, here comes another gene called **APOE**, which plays a role in keeping our brains and hearts healthy. But when there's a mix-up in this gene, it can lead to some tricky situations, like **Alzheimer's disease** or problems with our heart's highways called arteries.

But wait, there's a gene party happening in our **Mitochondria** too!

These genes decide how much energy we have, and if there's a special mutation, it might even help us live to be super old, like past 100!

Now, let's talk about **Blood pressure**, the force that keeps our blood flowing smoothly through our bodies.

Genes like AGT, ATE, and ATIR are like little switches that can influence how high or low our blood pressure goes.

But watch out for the **Pai-1** gene!

When it's not playing nice, it can cause our blood to get a bit too clingy, forming clots where they shouldn't be. But don't worry, if someone has this gene acting up, they can take a special potion called Pai-i to keep those clots at bay.

Finally, meet the **Enos** gene, our blood vessel wizard! It's responsible for making a magical substance called nitric oxide, which helps our blood vessels relax and stay flexible. But if there's a mutation in this gene, it could lead to some bumpy roads ahead, like **atherosclerosis**, where our arteries get all clogged up.

So, isn't it amazing how these **tiny genes** can make such a big difference in our bodies?

Keep exploring, little scientists! Who knows what other gene secrets are waiting to be discovered?

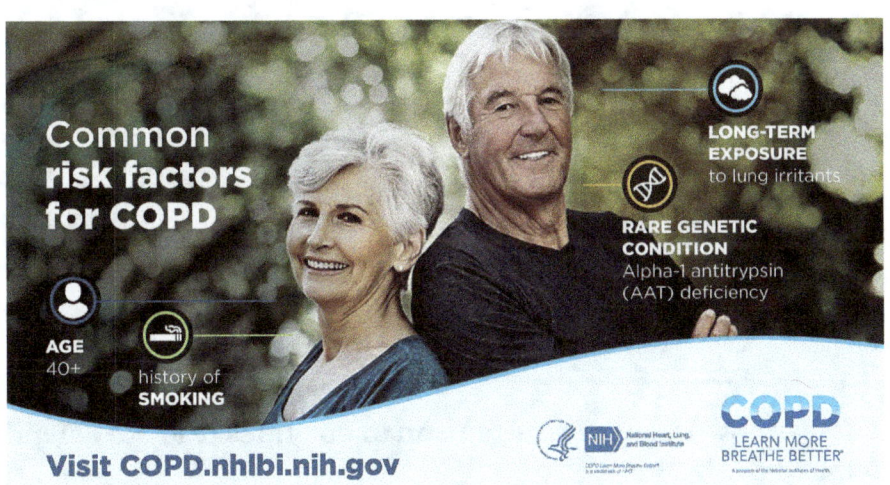

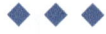

Single Nucleotide Polymorphism

Hey there, curious minds! Let's embark on a gene adventure and explore how our bodies handle all sorts of stuff, from toxins to medicines!

First up, we've got something called a **single nucleotide polymorphism**, or SNP for short. It's like a little switch in our genes that can affect how our bodies work.

Take **cytochrome P456-206**, for example.

It's a liver superhero that helps us detoxify yucky environmental toxins and break down medicines so they're safe for our bodies.

Now, here's a gene called **GSTM**. It's like a shield against the bad guys but get this—about half of the folks with lighter skin, called Caucasians, are born without it!

That means they might be more likely to get a visit from the **big C word, cancer**. But if you're lucky enough to have this gene in tip-top shape, it helps keep those environmental baddies at bay.

But fear not, because there's a **team of enzymes** ready to defend our bodies!

We've got GST MI, GSTP-1, CYPIAI, CYP-ib1, and CYP-2a6—they're like the Avengers of detoxification, swooping in to protect us from those pesky toxins.

Now, let's talk about the **CEPT gene**. If you've got a little hiccup in at least one of these genes from one of your parents, it might mean trouble for your "good" **cholesterol**, called HDL.

And you know what? HDL is like the bodyguard for your heart, so if it's not doing its job, it could mean a higher chance of having a heart attack.

So, there you have it, Youngsters!

Our genes are like our own personal superheroes, working hard to keep us safe and sound.

Keep exploring, and who knows what other gene mysteries we'll uncover!

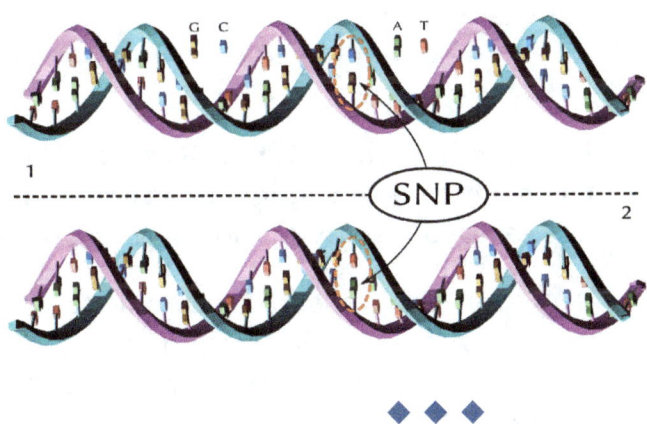

♦ ♦ ♦

Alrighty, let's make learning about our bodies a blast!

Meet **Familial Juvenile Polyposis**, or FJP for short! It's like a tricky puzzle game happening on loci 18g and 10g, where two genes called SMAD4 and BMPR1A are at play.

But watch out! If these genes don't work right, it can lead to a big showdown with a scary thing called colorectal cancer. But don't worry, with the right treatment, we can beat this villain!

Next up, say hello to **Down's syndrome**! It's like having an extra special chromosome 21 in our body, and it makes us unique in our awesome way!

Now, let's talk about Testicular Carcinoma. It's like a sneaky ninja hiding in our bodies. But fear not, we've got tools like HCG, Alpha-feto-protein, and Lactate dehydrogenase to help us spot and fight this ninja off!

Oh, and check out **Insulinoma** Tumors! They're like little troublemakers causing mischief in our bodies. But with a somatic mutation in the YY1 gene, we can kick these troublemakers to the curb!

Now, buckle up for **Antiphospholipid Antibody Syndrome**! It's like a rollercoaster ride in our blood, making it extra sticky. But we've got tricks up our sleeves to keep things flowing smoothly!

Zooming into the 42 AFI mutation, it's like a wild adventure leading us to chronic myelocytic leukemia. But with heroes like Thyroid transcription factor-1 and TTR, we're ready to tackle anything that comes our way!

And who could forget about GST genotype D? It's like having a secret weapon against toxins!

Finally, let's give a round of applause to TP53! It's like the guardian of our cells, making sure they stay good guys. Without it, those cells might turn rogue and cause trouble!

So, there you have it, Youngsters!

Our bodies are like action-packed adventures filled with heroes, villains, and all sorts of surprises.

Keep exploring and learning, and remember, you're the superhero of your own story!

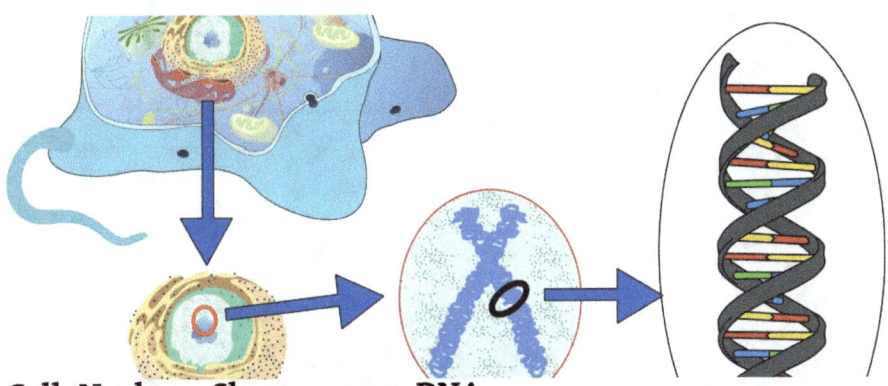

Cell- Nucleus- Chromosome- DNA

◆ ◆ ◆

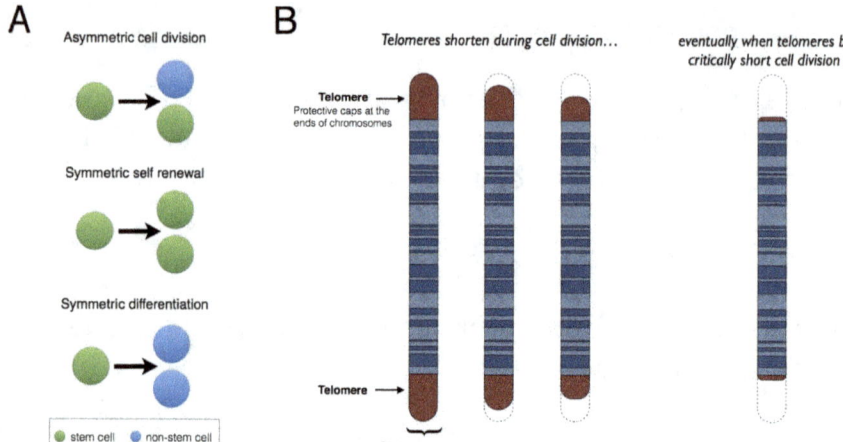

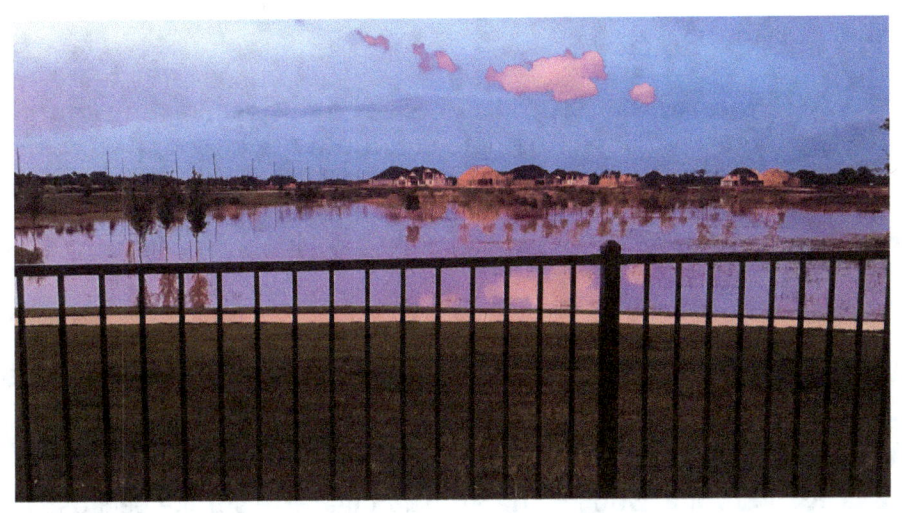

CHAPTER 7

Environmental DNA Damagers

Eco Tips for All

Hey youngsters! Let's talk about some sneaky stuff out there called Environmental DNA Damagers!

But don't worry, we've got some super cool ways to avoid them!

1. Underarm Deodorant: Swap out those smelly ones for something supernatural like cornstarch and baking soda! It's like magic for your armpits!

2. Shower Soap: Instead of soaps with weird ingredients, try ones made with olive oil and minerals. Check out the organic websites for cool recipes!

3. Watch out for Bad Stuff: Say no-no to things like aluminum, parabens, and PHTH toxins. They're not invited to our party!

4. Pesky Pesticides: Eating organic plants and animals helps keep away those nasty pesticides. They're like the bullies of the garden!

5. Tricky Chemicals: Stay away from things like organohalides found in pesticides and soil degreasers. They're like the villains in a superhero movie!

6. Yucky Smoke: Don't hang around cigarette smoke because it has icky things called aromatic amines that can make you sick.

7. Plastic Problems: Avoid using plastic bottles and fast food containers, especially in the microwave. They can have sneaky chemicals like PCBs that we don't want near us!

8. Heavy Metals: Lead, cadmium, and mercury are like the bad guys in a video game. We don't want them in our bodies!

9. Air and Water Woes: Watch out for environmental toxins in the air and water, like pollution and radon. They're like invisible monsters!

10. Colorful Caution: Be careful with colorful dyes like red dye 40 and yellow dye 5. They might look fun, but they're not good for us.

11. No Toxins Allowed: Say goodbye to antibacterial soaps. They might sound helpful, but they're full of yucky toxins.

Remember, by being smart and choosing the right stuff, we can keep those Environmental DNA Damagers far, far away!

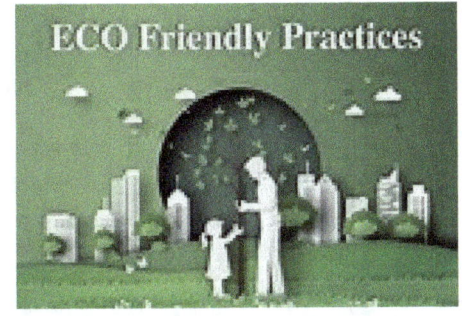

Carcinogens.

Hey there, Youngsters!
Let's talk about some sneaky stuff called Carcinogens that can mess with our Environmental DNA! But don't worry, we've got some superhero tips to keep them at bay!

1. Watch Out for Tricky Triclosan: Stay away from products with a bad guy called Triclosan. It's like a ninja that can harm our DNA!

2. Bye-bye to Aluminum and Mercury: Say no to aluminum and mercury fillings in your teeth. They're like the villains of our smiles!

3. Deodorants without Aluminum: Pick deodorants without aluminum. It's like choosing a superhero cape that keeps us safe and fresh!

4. Dye Danger: Be cautious with colorful dyes like red dye 40, yellow dye 5, and blue dye. They might look fun, but they're not good for our bodies!

5. Radon Rocks: Radon in homes can be sneaky, causing lung cancer. Let's make sure our homes are radon-free!

6. Beware of Rays: UV light, X-rays, and gamma rays might sound cool, but they're like sneaky villains that can cause cancer. Let's stay away from them!

7. Fishy Business: Be careful with fish because some of them can have mercury, PCBs, and other yucky stuff. Let's pick our fishy friends wisely!

8. Check the List: The CDC has a list of known carcinogens. Let's check it out to know what to avoid!

9. Plastic Problems: Plastic shower curtains can be tricky. They might look harmless, but they can cause cancer. Let's find safer alternatives!

10. Building Safety: Visit websites like EPA and NSC to learn about building safety. They're like our superhero headquarters for staying healthy!

11. Vitamin Heroes: Make sure to get enough vitamins like B6, B12, C, folic acid, iron, and zinc. They're like our superhero sidekicks, protecting us from DNA damage and cancer!

Remember, with our superhero knowledge, we can defeat those sneaky Carcinogens and keep our DNA safe and sound!
EPA-sick building - www.epa.gov/reg/puba/at.
NSC- National Safety Council - www.nk.org/ech/sbs.html

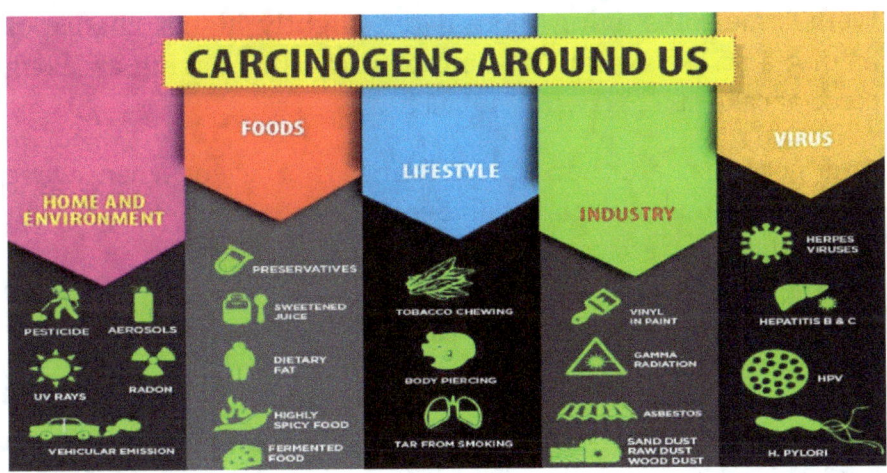

Airport Noise

Hey, Youngsters!
Let's chat about something really interesting and a bit funny too – Airport Noise!

Did you know that living near noisy airports can sometimes cause heart problems?

Yup, it's true! But don't worry, we've got the scoop on what's going on.

So, picture this: Imagine you're living near a super busy airport like the one in Germany called Frankfurt.

Well, some folks living there had a slightly higher chance of having a stroke – about 7% more! That's like having an extra piece of cake at a party, but not as fun.

And get this, another study found that even when we're snoozing, those airplane flyovers near Zurich airport in Switzerland can affect our hearts!

Yup, nighttime can be noisy too, especially when planes are zooming by.

Now, let's talk about what happens in our bodies when we hear loud noises. It's like our brains hit the panic button!

Our blood pressure goes up, hormones start doing a crazy dance, and some of our arteries get all twisty and turn. It's like a big party in our bodies, but not the fun kind!

According to a smart guy named Mathias Basner, who knows a lot about this stuff, all this noise can mess with something called the endothelium – which is like the cozy blanket lining our blood vessels.

When it gets inflamed, it's like a grumpy cat, making things a bit tricky for our blood to flow smoothly. And guess what? Even just a few nights of loud airplane noise can make it act up!

So, next time you hear a loud plane, just remember, it's not just noise – it's like a mini adventure for our bodies too!

But don't worry, with some earplugs and maybe a bedtime story, we'll keep those airplane noises at bay and our hearts happy!

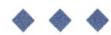

Cool CRISPR Cancer Fight!

Clustered Regularly Interspaced Short Palindromic Repeat Clinical.trials.gov.Crispr.

Hey youngsters! Let's talk about CRISPR, a super cool tool scientists use to edit genes in our bodies.

Imagine your body is like a big instruction book, called DNA. CRISPR is like a special pair of scissors that can cut this book at specific places.

CRISPR has a helper called Cas-9, which is like a ninja. It helps CRISPR find and destroy certain parts of the instructions in our DNA.

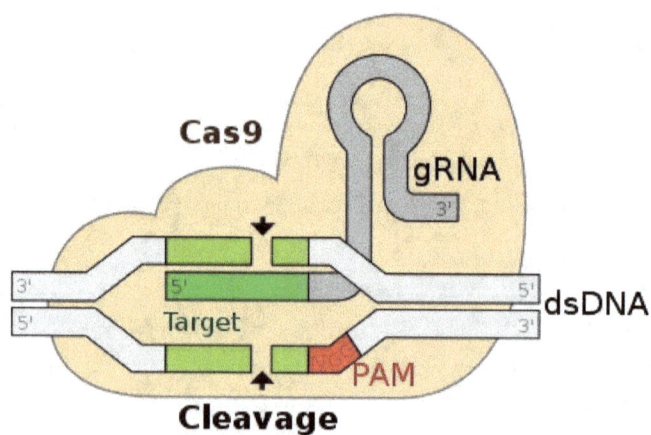

Now, let's talk about some other ways we're fighting against diseases like cancer!

Have you heard of Car-T?

It's like giving your body's soldiers, called **T-cells**, superpowers to fight cancer. Scientists modify these T-cells and send them back into your body to fight off those pesky cancer cells.

Then, there are **vaccines**. They work like shields, helping our bodies recognize and attack cancer cells.

Another cool way to fight diseases is through **epigenetic reprogramming**. Think of it like soothing music for our cells. It helps relax our bodies and makes them stronger to fight against diseases.

So, whether it's using CRISPR scissors, giving T-cells superpowers, using vaccines as shields, or relaxing with music therapy, scientists are always finding new ways to help us stay healthy and strong!

IMMUNOTHERAPY FOR LUNG AND OTHER CANCERS

IMMUNOTHERAPIES CALLED CHECKPOINT INHIBITORS are changing the landscape of treatment for lung, melanoma and other cancers. Several approved immunotherapies inhibit the PD-1/PD-L1 cell signaling pathway, and one inhibits the CTLA-4 pathway. All of these drugs work by taking the brakes off the immune system and boosting its power to fight cancer.

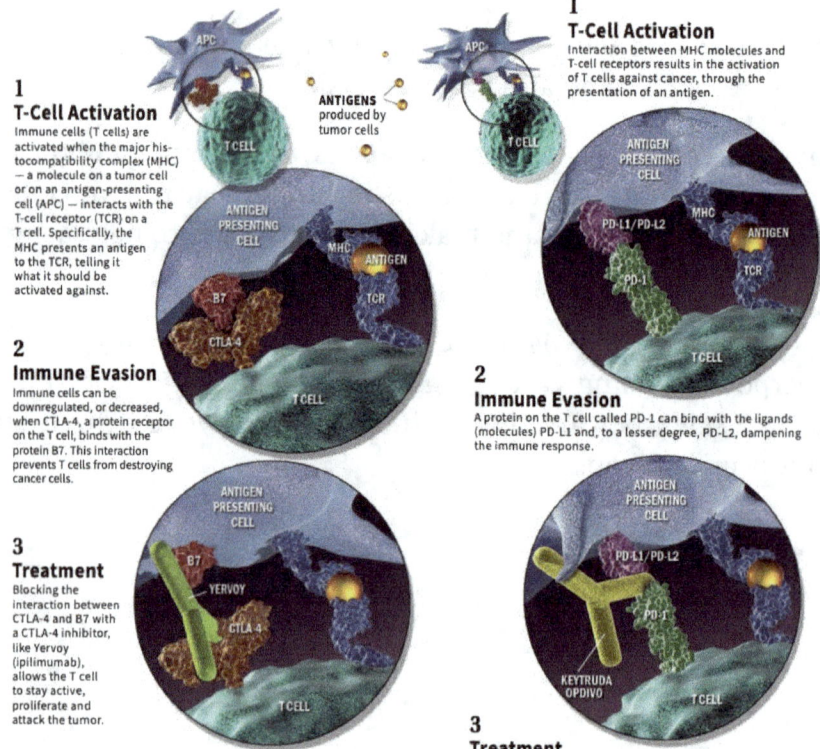

CTLA-4 Pathway

1 T-Cell Activation
Immune cells (T cells) are activated when the major histocompatibility complex (MHC) — a molecule on a tumor cell or on an antigen-presenting cell (APC) — interacts with the T-cell receptor (TCR) on a T cell. Specifically, the MHC presents an antigen to the TCR, telling it what it should be activated against.

2 Immune Evasion
Immune cells can be downregulated, or decreased, when CTLA-4, a protein receptor on the T cell, binds with the protein B7. This interaction prevents T cells from destroying cancer cells.

3 Treatment
Blocking the interaction between CTLA-4 and B7 with a CTLA-4 inhibitor, like Yervoy (ipilimumab), allows the T cell to stay active, proliferate and attack the tumor.

PD-1/PD-L1 Pathway

1 T-Cell Activation
Interaction between MHC molecules and T-cell receptors results in the activation of T cells against cancer, through the presentation of an antigen.

2 Immune Evasion
A protein on the T cell called PD-1 can bind with the ligands (molecules) PD-L1 and, to a lesser degree, PD-L2, dampening the immune response.

3 Treatment
Blocking PD-1 or PD-L1 with Keytruda (pembrolizumab), Opdivo (nivolumab), Tecentriq (atezolizumab), Imfinzi (durvalumab) or Bavencio (avelumab) allows the T cells to remain activated against the tumor.

ANTIGENS produced by tumor cells

CAR-T CELL THERAPY

CHIMERIC ANTIGEN RECEPTOR (CAR)-T cell therapy is a form of immunotherapy. This laboratory-assisted method modifies a patient's own immune cells to fight cancer that has developed in the body.

The therapy involves removing a patient's T cells and "engineering" them to recognize and attack a cancer-specific antigen, or molecule, on the surface of cancer cells. A genetic sequence is inserted into the T cells, causing them to develop receptors capable of binding to the antigens on cancer cells. Binding triggers the T cells to destroy the malignant cells.

Two CAR-T cell therapies have been approved by the Food and Drug Administration: Kymriah (tisagenlecleucel) and Yescarta (axicabtagene ciloleucel) for acute lymphoblastic leukemia and non-Hodgkin lymphoma, respectively. These drugs target the antigen CD19 that sits on cancer cells associated with those malignancies. In addition, scientists are testing CAR-T cell therapies that target the antigen BCMA on multiple myeloma cells.

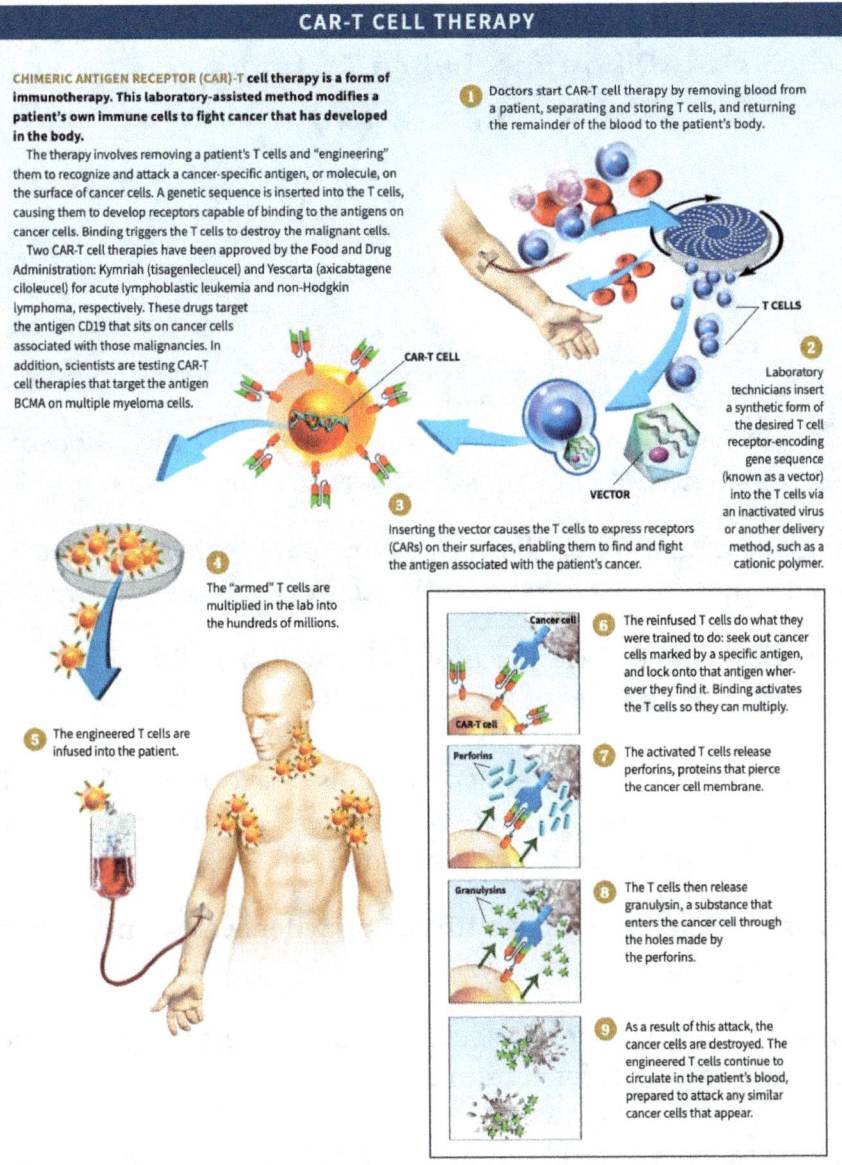

1. Doctors start CAR-T cell therapy by removing blood from a patient, separating and storing T cells, and returning the remainder of the blood to the patient's body.

2. Laboratory technicians insert a synthetic form of the desired T cell receptor-encoding gene sequence (known as a vector) into the T cells via an inactivated virus or another delivery method, such as a cationic polymer.

3. Inserting the vector causes the T cells to express receptors (CARs) on their surfaces, enabling them to find and fight the antigen associated with the patient's cancer.

4. The "armed" T cells are multiplied in the lab into the hundreds of millions.

5. The engineered T cells are infused into the patient.

6. The reinfused T cells do what they were trained to do: seek out cancer cells marked by a specific antigen, and lock onto that antigen wherever they find it. Binding activates the T cells so they can multiply.

7. The activated T cells release perforins, proteins that pierce the cancer cell membrane.

8. The T cells then release granulysin, a substance that enters the cancer cell through the holes made by the perforins.

9. As a result of this attack, the cancer cells are destroyed. The engineered T cells continue to circulate in the patient's blood, prepared to attack any similar cancer cells that appear.

Ribosome Switch Technology (Riboswitch)

Hey there, Youngsters! Let's talk about something super cool called Ribosome Switch Technology, or Riboswitch for short!

Imagine a Riboswitch like a tiny controller inside our cells. It's like a remote control that helps us turn certain genes on and off.

Scientists put a little piece of RNA, which is like a message carrier, into the genes of a patient's cells.

Then, they give the patient special pills or eye drops. These pills or drops help close the Riboswitch, like shutting a door, which allows the new genes to start working.

The switched genes can be turned on whenever we need them, like every hour or every day.

This amazing technology helps control gene therapies, which are like treatments for certain illnesses.

It can also help control things like insulin or other hormones in our bodies.

So, think of Riboswitch as our body's little switchboard, helping us stay healthy and strong!

Cool, right?

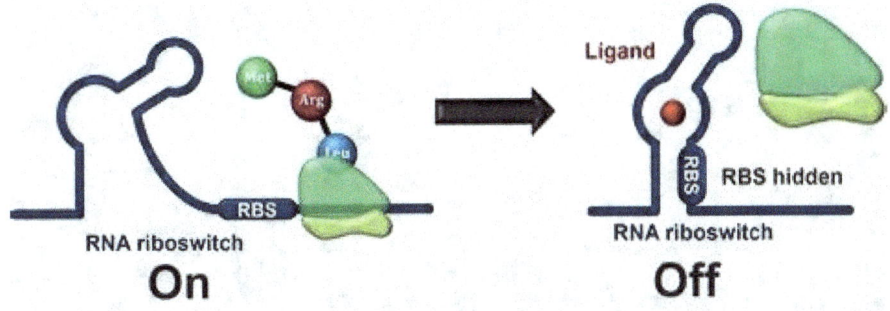

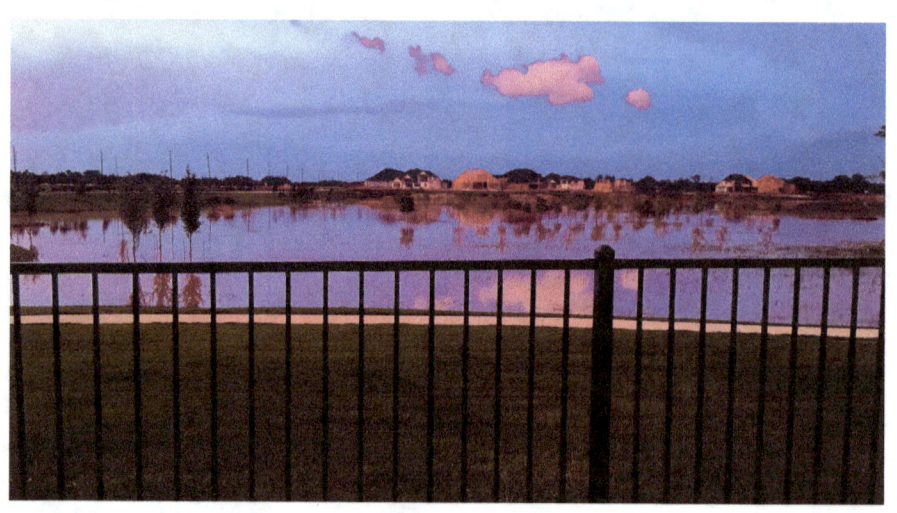

CHAPTER 8

Dementia: Mini-Mental-State Summary

Simplified version of the Mini-Mental State Examination:

1. Orientation Test:

What's today's date?

Where are we (city, state)?

What's your name?

Can you name a family member?

2. Attention Test:

Repeat a short list of objects (like black hat, red shoe, 42nd street).

3. Immediate Recall:

Repeat the objects mentioned earlier after three minutes.

4. Recent Memory Test:

Recall an event from a few days ago (like what you had for lunch on Wednesday or Friday).

5. Remote Memory Test:

Recall past events like wedding anniversaries or birthdays.

6. Abstract Thinking Test:

Explain the meaning of a proverb, for example, "A rolling stone gathers no moss".

7. Insight into Illness/Dementia:

Share your feelings and opinions about dementia.

8. Mood Test:

How do you feel today?

How do you usually feel?

9. Fund of Knowledge Test:

Name the last five presidents or state capitals.

10. Ability to Follow Simple Commands:

Follow instructions like putting your right thumb over your left ear and sticking out your tongue.

11. Ability to Use Language:

Name body parts and read, write, and repeat phrases like "cool one another".

12. Ability to Process Sensory Information:

Identify objects placed in your hand with your eyes closed.

Recognize a number drawn on your palm.

Differentiate between touch sensations on your palm and fingers with your eyes closed.

13. Spatial Relationships Test:

Draw a clock.

Draw cubes.

Draw two intersecting cubes.

14. Ability to Perform Tasks:

Demonstrate how you brush your teeth.

15. Math Problem Solving:

Solve simple math problems like 9 times 5 equals 45, 8 times 8 equals 64, and 72 divided by 12 equals 6.

LIVE LONGER LOVE LONGER PART 3

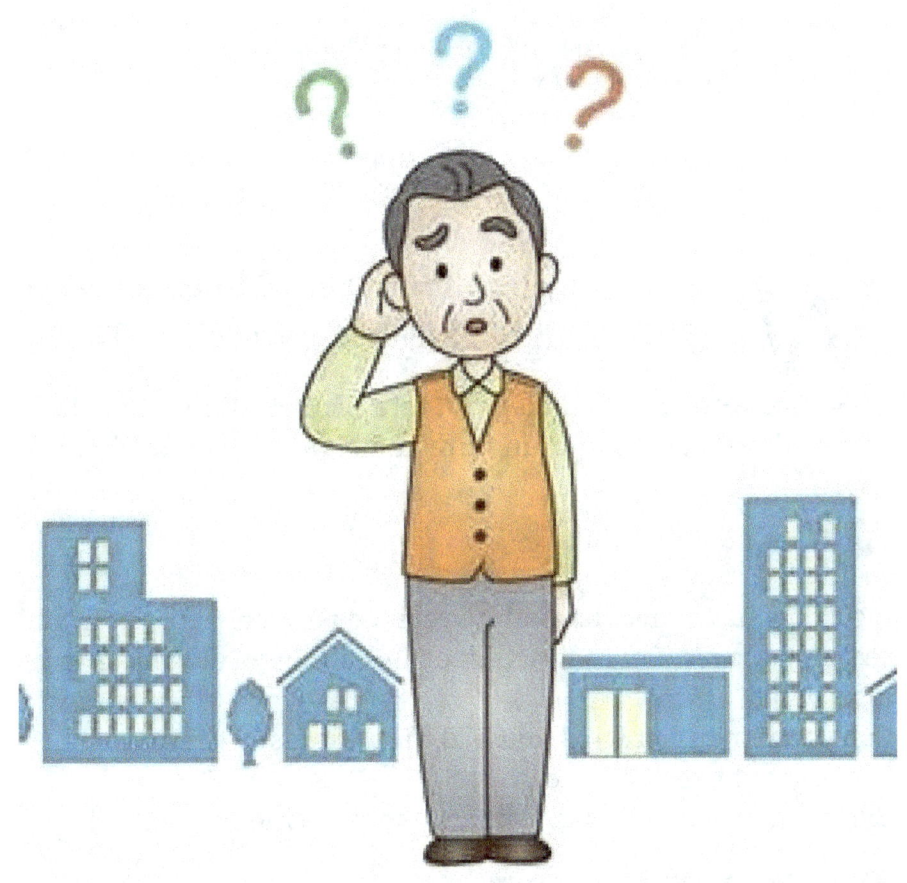

Title: Fun Brain Quiz Adventure!

Welcome to the Fun Brain Quiz Adventure! Are you ready to embark on a journey through your mind? Let's dive into the Mini-Mental-State Examination – but don't worry, there's nothing miniature about the fun we're about to have!

Step 1: The Memory Maze

Picture yourself in a magical maze filled with colorful doors and secret passages. Behind each door lies a memory waiting to be discovered!
Can you remember what you had for breakfast yesterday?
What about your favorite color?
Explore the maze and unlock the memories hidden within!

Step 2: Counting Conundrum

Next, let's test those counting skills! Imagine you're a treasure hunter on a quest to find the lost coins.
But beware – the coins are scattered all over the place, and you must count them as fast as you can before they disappear!
Ready, set, count!

Step 3: Shape Shifter Challenge

Now, let's get creative with shapes!

Picture yourself as a master artist, sculpting clay into all sorts of wacky shapes and figures.
Can you identify the square, circle, and triangle?

Get ready to mold your mind into shape-shifting perfection!

Step 4: Word Wonderland

Ahoy, mateys! It's time to set sail on World Wonderland!

Imagine you're a brave explorer navigating through a sea of words.
Can you name objects beginning with the letter "B"? How about naming as many animals as you can in one minute?
Let your imagination run wild as you conquer the Word Wonderland!

Step 5: Storybook Challenge

Last but not least, let's put your storytelling skills to the test!

Picture yourself as the hero of your very own storybook adventure. Can you recount a favorite tale from beginning to end? Use your creativity and imagination to bring the story to life!

Congratulations, adventurer!
You've completed the Fun Brain Quiz Adventure and unlocked the secrets of your mind!
Now go forth and explore the wonders of your imagination – the possibilities are endless!

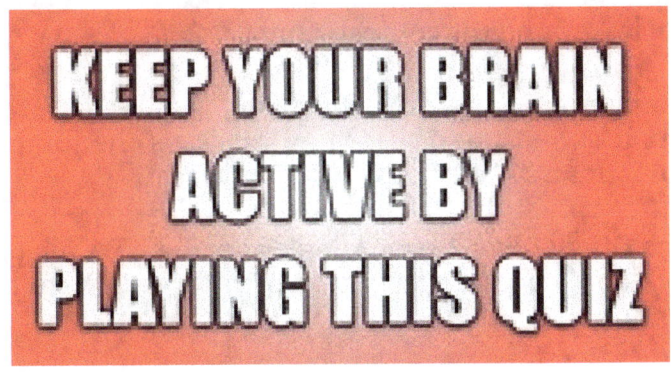

For Brain Power Over 60 Years of Age

Alright, let's sprinkle some humor onto these brain-boosting tips for the over-60 crowd:

1. Espresso Expedition: Who needs a map when you've got espresso? With 2-3 cups a day, you'll be zipping through the day faster than a caffeine-fueled rocket!

2. Intermittent Hilarity: Forget about counting calories, let's count the hours until our next meal! Intermittent fasting – because who doesn't love a little hunger-induced comedy?

3. Snooze Cruise: Ah, the sweet sound of snoring after a 3-mile stroll. If you're an elite athlete, make sure to book a 10-hour ticket to Sleep City – population: you, catching Z's like a champ!

4. Fishy Brain Treats: Want to be as sharp as a swordfish? Dive into some omega-3 fatty acids from fish oil and watch your brain swim circles around the competition!

5. Choco mania: Forget milk chocolate, it's all about that dark chocolate life! 500 mg of cocoa a day keeps the forgetfulness away – plus, it's a sweet excuse for a daily treat!

6. Ginkgo Giggle-oba: Prevent dementia and have a laugh with Ginkgo biloba – because who wants to forget where they left their dentures?

7. Statin Stories: Zocor, the superhero of medications! Not only does it fight off colon and prostate cancer like a boss, but it also takes Alzheimer's disease on a slow, leisurely stroll. Talk about multitasking!

8. Pill Pals: Who knew Viagra and Cialis were the ultimate wingman for your brain? Just remember, consult your doctor before inviting them to the party!

9. Hormonal High Jinks: Testosterone and human growth hormone replacement – because who says aging can't be an adventure?

10. Acetyl-l-carnitine Amusement: Say that five times fast! This brain-booster is your ticket to memory lane – just don't forget where you parked!

11. Vinpocetine Voyage: Ahoy, mateys! Set sail with Vinpocetine and watch as your brain's blood flow becomes smoother than a pirate's silk scarf!

12. Nexrutine Nonsense: What's the deal with Nexrutine? Nobody knows, but it's in the brain game, so it must be good, right?

13. Quirky Quercetin: Quercetin – because who doesn't love a good tongue twister before bed?

14. Pregnenolone Party: Pregnenolone – the life of the brain party! Just don't let it hog all the spotlights.

15. Modafinil Madness: Need a pick-me-up? Modafinil's got you covered – just be prepared for some seriously enhanced cognitive hijinks!

16. Donepezil Drama: Slow down memory loss with Donepezil – because who needs a fast-paced brain when you can take it easy?

17. Brainy Business: Age-associated memory impairment – it's like a crossword puzzle for your brain! Keep it active with books, newspapers, and intellectual activities – because who needs brain fog when you can have a brainstorm?

18. Viagra Vibes: Feeling the love? Thank Viagra for that oxytocin boost – who knew a little blue pill could lead to a brainy romance?

So there you have it, folks – brain power over 60, served with a side of laughter!

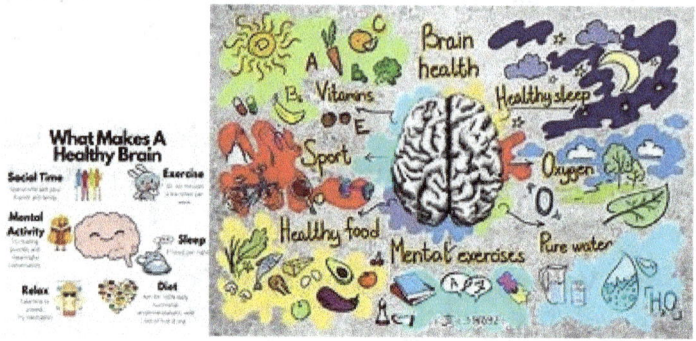

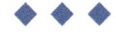

Behavioral Variant Frontotemporal Dementia

Let's make this information more kid-friendly and easier to understand:

1. Feeling Forgetful: People with this kind of dementia might have trouble understanding others' feelings, acting appropriately in social situations, or thinking in creative ways.

2. Funny Behaviors: Sometimes they might do silly or strange things without thinking, like acting on impulses or getting stuck doing the same thing over and over.

They might also not seem very interested in things they used to enjoy, except maybe for sweet treats or foods that are not so good for them.

3. Memory Mystery: Surprisingly, their memory might stay pretty good compared to other types of dementia.

4. Brain Changes: Doctors can see changes in a part of the brain called the frontal lobe. It's like a muscle that's not working right in this kind of dementia.

5. Weird Protein: Inside their brain cells, there's a funny protein that builds up and makes things go wrong. It's like having too many toys cluttering up a room!

6. Super Science Stuff: Sometimes, there are mistakes in their genes, kind of like typos in a book. These mistakes can make them more likely to have this kind of dementia.

7. Thinking Troubles: Their brain might not work as quickly or as well as it used to. They might find it hard to focus, plan, or make good decisions.

8. Feeling Meh: Even though they might not seem sad, they might just not care about things as much as they used to. It's like feeling "blah" about everything.

So, youngsters, remember to be patient and understanding with people who have these changes in their brains.

They might act a bit differently, but they're still the same person inside!

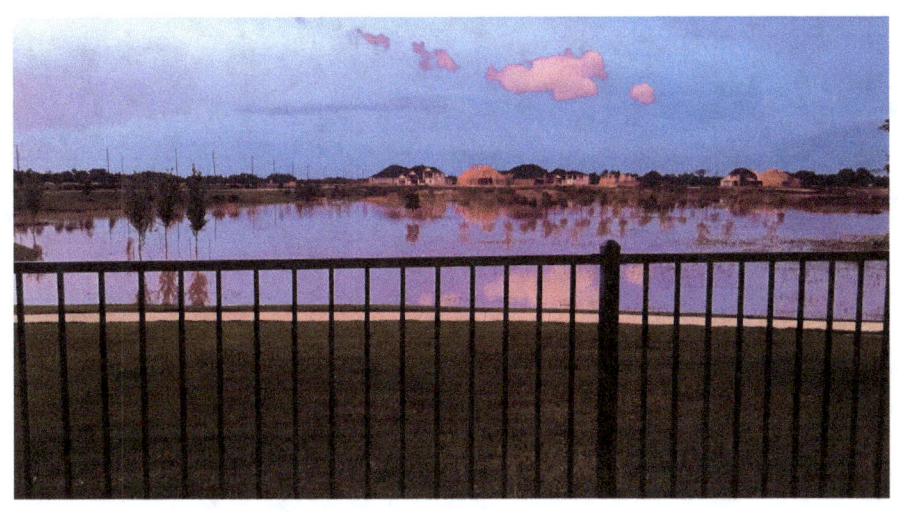

CHAPTER 9

Breakthrough Technology

L et's simplify the information for better understanding:

Imagine wearing a special cap that sends gentle pulses to different parts of your brain. When these pulses target the back part of your brain, called the parietal cortex, they help you remember words better, especially those at the end of a list.

But wait, there's more!

When the pulses target the front part of your brain, called the prefrontal cortex, they boost your memory for words at the beginning of a list.

This treatment works by changing how fast your brain cells communicate with each other and encourages your brain to adapt and form new connections, kind of like training your brain to be more efficient.

The cool part?

It helps improve your memory for a short while, but the effects fade once the treatment stops.

So, it's like giving your brain a little workout session to enhance your memory skills!

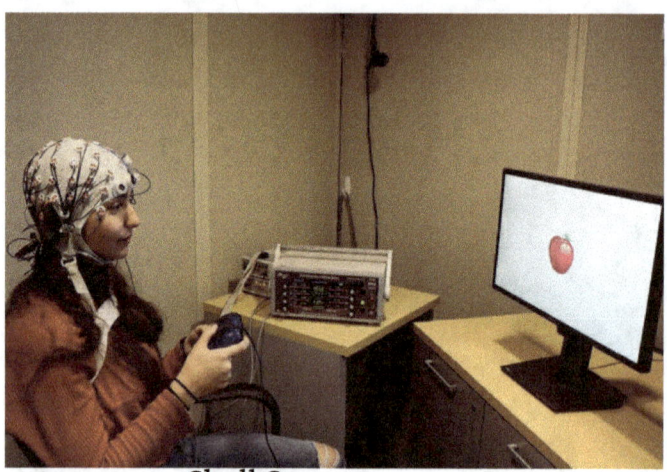

Skull Cap

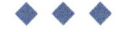

Innovative Technologies

Let's break down these innovative technologies in simpler terms:

1. **Quellbre:** a non-stimulant that Helps manage ADHD symptoms.

2. **Ocrevus**: Treats multiple sclerosis twice a year.

3. **Vraylar**: A treatment for bipolar type 1 disorder.

4. **Leqvio**: Lowers cholesterol with just two doses per year.

5. **Oncotype dx**: Helps doctors choose the best chemotherapy for cancer.

6. **Transcranial Magnetic Stimulation (TMS)**: Treats depression, drug addiction, cigarette addiction, and alcohol addiction by stimulating the brain.

7. **Cepheid Medical Office PCR Machine**: Tests for Influenza A&B, Sars-Cov-2, and RSV using nasal swabs.

8. **BioFire Diagnostics Respiratory Test**: Identifies 17 viruses and three bacteria from a single nasal swab in just 30 minutes.

9. **Aveyo Technologies**: Offers a handheld molecular testing machine with results in 30 minutes.

10. **Visby Medical Device**: Tests for chlamydia, gonorrhea, and

Sars-Cov-2.

11. **Ascencio Dx**: Detects HIV and ELU, with a rapid molecular Covid test.

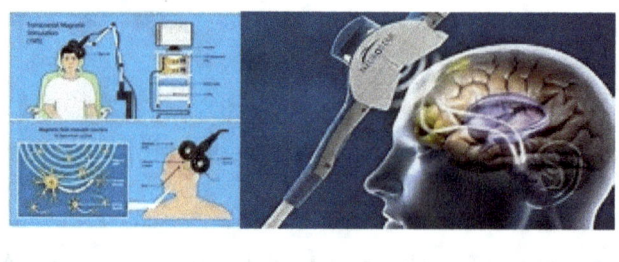

◆ ◆ ◆

Aging Technologies Revolution

Revolutionary Technologies Targeting Aging: A Continued Exploration

1. Vision Enhancement through Utility Eye Drops: These drops work to reduce pupil size, enhancing near-vision clarity and potentially eliminating the need for reading glasses.

2. mRNA Therapy: Mayo Clinic has pioneered the use of mRNA technology to bolster the body's T-cell response, effectively combating cancer, particularly advanced melanoma.

The five-year survival rate has soared from a mere 5% a decade ago to an impressive 50% today.

3. AI-driven Oculomics for Disease Prediction: Leveraging artificial intelligence, this breakthrough technology analyzes eye scans to predict cardiovascular diseases based on retinal artery conditions.

Its future applications extend to forecasting neurological ailments like Alzheimer's disease, multiple sclerosis, Parkinson's disease, and stroke.

4. Smart Contact Lenses by Allure Thera Vision: These innovative lenses release antihistamines to alleviate allergy-induced eye itching.

Moreover, ongoing research aims to equip these lenses with features to enhance athletic performance, providing real-time insights and guidance.

These advancements stand at the forefront of combating age-related health issues, offering promising solutions to improve quality of life and longevity.

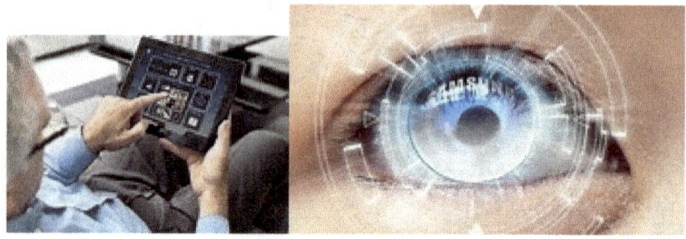

Conatct lense with Camera.

Riboswitch

Meira GTX Holdings has developed a remarkable technology called Riboswitch, which acts as a regulatory switch controlling artificial gene therapy within a patient's cells.

1. It targets a condition called Familial **Hypercholesterolemia**, where high cholesterol runs in families due to a specific genetic mutation.

Meira's Riboswitch intervenes by addressing antibodies that attack a key protein responsible for regulating cholesterol levels, offering a potential treatment for this condition.

2. Additionally, this technology shows promise in treating inherited eye diseases by regulating genes associated with vision health.

3. Meira's Riboswitch also plays a role in regulating the gene responsible for producing **erythropoietin**, a hormone that stimulates the production of red blood cells.

4. Looking ahead, Riboswitches hold the potential to control **gene therapies** for various conditions like Hemophilia and Parkinson's disease, offering new avenues for treatment.

5. Moreover, Riboswitches could be utilized to regulate insulin production, potentially offering a novel approach to managing diabetes.

They might also be placed in the brain to treat conditions

like brain cancer or neurodegenerative diseases by controlling specific molecules that can cross the protective barrier surrounding the brain.

Incredible Breakthroughs in Healthcare!

1. Inspire Implant for Sleep Apnea: A game-changing solution for **sleep apnea**, this implant, known as CPAP/BIPAP Inspire, offers relief by effectively regulating breathing during sleep.

2. Rinvoq: This groundbreaking treatment revolutionizes the management of **eczema**, providing effective relief for sufferers.

3. Quviq: Say goodbye to sleepless nights with Quviq, a cutting-edge treatment designed to combat **insomnia** and promote restful sleep.

4. Leqvio: Offering convenience and effectiveness, Leqvio presents a two-dose injection per year to effectively lower **cholesterol** levels.

5. Lume: Banish **body odor** woes with Lume, an over-the-counter solution providing 12-hour relief from unpleasant odors, including "butt stink."

6. Uqora: Providing swift relief, Uqura offers an over-the-counter treatment for **urinary tract infections**, offering convenience and efficacy.

7. Advanced Lasik Eye Surgery: Transforming vision correction, Lasik eye surgery now offers solutions for both near and far **vision**, with the option of lens implants if needed, providing clarity without glasses or contacts.

8. Cutting-Edge Hearing Aids: Experience enhanced hearing with the latest advancements in hearing aid technology, offering improved **sound** quality and comfort.

INSPIRE UPPER AIRWAY STIMULATION (UAS) THERAPY

Stimulation of the upper airway prevents airway collapse during breathing

Sensor detects each time patient breathes

Stimulation

Airway maintained open during therapy

Pulse generator processes breathing data and provides stimulation

◆ ◆ ◆

Platelet-Rich Plasma (PRP) Therapy

PRP therapy harnesses the body's natural healing capabilities to address conditions such as lateral and medial epicondylitis (commonly known as tennis elbow and golfer's elbow) as well as knee arthritis.

Here's how it works:

1. A kit containing Platelet-Rich Plasma (PRP) solution is prepared, typically priced at $175 per kit, which is then

administered at a charge of $1200.

2. The PRP solution consists of 50 cc, along with a 10 cc anticoagulant, ensuring optimal efficacy.

3. The process involves spinning the solution twice to concentrate platelets and growth factors before injecting it directly into the affected joint.

4. PRP therapy has shown significant efficacy in treating conditions like tennis elbow, golfer's elbow, and tendon degeneration. Studies have indicated a remarkable 71.5% improvement in pain scores after 24 weeks compared to 56.1% in the control group.

5. Moreover, for patients suffering from knee osteoarthritis, PRP therapy has demonstrated superior pain reduction compared to placebo and hyaluronic acid injections, with success rates reaching 78% versus 74%.

Platelet-rich plasma therapy offers a promising avenue for individuals seeking non-surgical solutions to alleviate pain and promote healing in various orthopedic conditions.

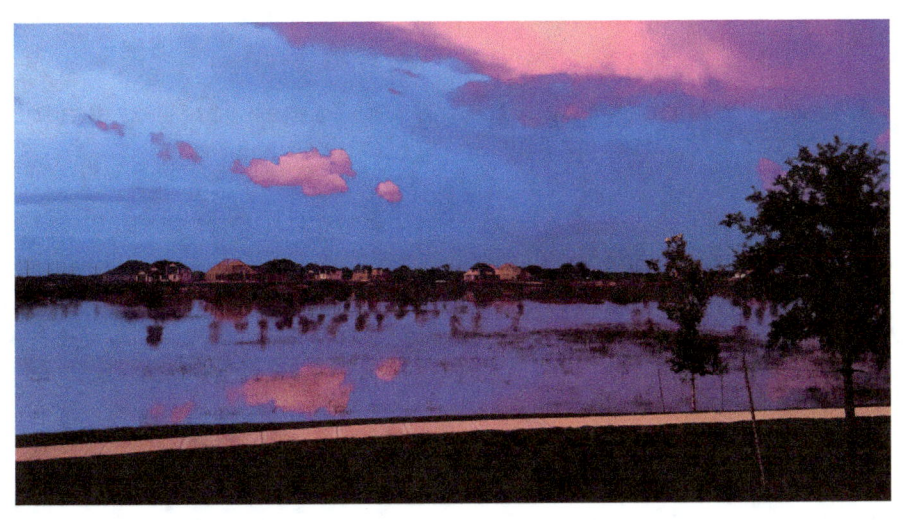

CHAPTER 10

*Breakthrough Medication:
Revolutionary Anti-aging
Medication Treatment Unveiled!*

Imbruvica: A Non-Chemotherapy Breakthrough for Chronic Lymphocytic Leukemia (CLL).

Carbenia: Bi-Monthly Game-Changer in HIV (AIDS) Treatment.

Circuit Clinical: Pioneering Traditional and Virtual Clinical Trials, Ensuring Inclusivity in Diverse Communities.

The TAME Study: Investigating Metformin's Potential to Halt Aging in the Elderly.

Aricept and Namenda: Leading the Charge Against Alzheimer's

Disease.

ALZ.org: Providing Support and Resources for Alzheimer's Patients and Families at Any Given Moment.

HCG/Testosterone Therapy: A Promising Approach to Rejuvenating Aging Bodies.

Viagra/Cialis: Transforming Lives Through Enhanced Sexual Health.

Stem Cells: Unlocking the Fountain of Youth Through Regenerative Medicine.

Platelet-Rich Plasma: Offering Relief Through Joint Injections for Degenerative Conditions.

Bioengineered RNA: A Cutting-Edge Intervention in Anti-Aging Research.

Ocrevus: Biannual Breakthrough for Multiple Sclerosis Management.

Mayret: Eight Weeks to Combat Hepatitis C and Restore Health.

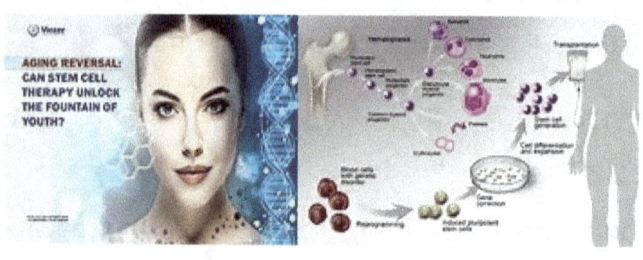

◆ ◆ ◆

Introducing the Laugh-Out-Loud Breakthrough Medications!

Pfizer presents **Tanezumab,** the "Ahhhhh" for Osteoarthritis

Pain Relief.

Rinvoq Upadacitinib: The Superhero Sidekick for Psoriatic Arthritis.

Prolia: Because Who Wants Osteoporosis When You Can Get a Six-Month Injection?

Lumify: Because Dry Eyes Are So Last Season - Blink, and You'll Not Miss the Relief!

Xofluza: The "No More Flu Boo-Hooza" Nasal Savior.

Kerasal: Putting the Fun Back in Fungal Treatment for Toes - Say Goodbye to Onychomycosis Blues!

L'oreal Revitalift: Fighting Wrinkles with Retinol, Because Who Says Aging Can't Be Comedy?

Libre Freestyle: Monitoring Glucose Levels Like A Pro - 24-Hour Skin Style!

Sono Bello: Sculpting Bodies and Bustling Bellies - Say Hello to the New You!

Genusil.com: Bye-Bye Jaw, Neck, Eye, and Crows Feet Woes - Creamier Than a Comedy Show!

Senolytics Biotin: Bidding Adieu to Senescent Cells - Because Age Is Just a Number, Not a Punchline!

And drumroll, please... Introducing the Brain Buster Breathe-in Treatment for Concussion - For Football Players and Other Head Bangers!

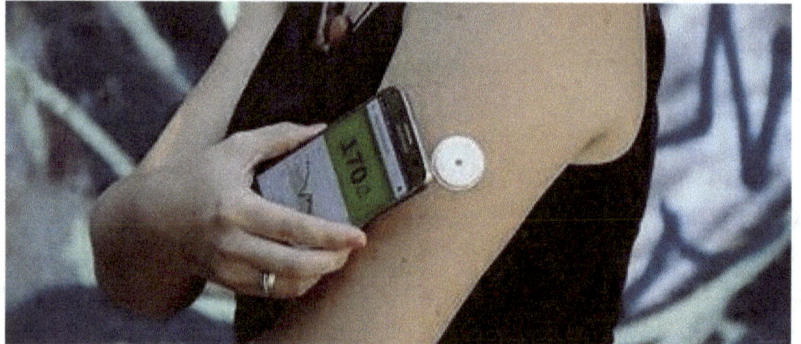

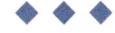

Reimagined!

Age-related Macular degeneration(AMD). Aging Eye Marvel Distress! Age-Related Eye Disease Studies (AREDS), Unveils Eye-Resting Delight! The secret to dodging (AMD) Age-Related Macular Downfall lies in a magical potion of multivitamin/mineral marvels!

Enter "**Preservision**" - not your ordinary eye elixir, but a wondrous ophthalmological prescription packed with vitamins, minerals, and a sprinkle of goodness from gluten, corn, leafy vegetables, and zeaxanthin.

Bid farewell to the evil Vitamin A, and welcome the era of eye-saving glory!

Source: EVANS J. R. et al. The Chronicles of Antioxidant Vitamin and Mineral Marvels: A Tale of Preventing Age-Related Macular Degeneration. Cochrane Database System Review, July 30, 2017; Volume 9, CD000253 [PMID 287566107].

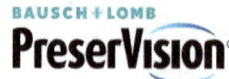

Explore Your Options

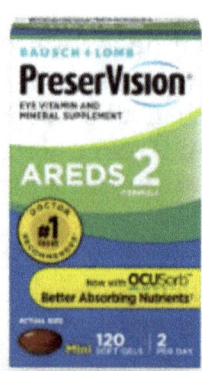

AREDS 2 Formula MiniGels

Contains the clinically proven AREDS 2 formula in a smaller pill.†

Stem Cell Therapy

Delving into the Revolutionary Realm of Stem Cell Therapy!

Consider Parkinson's Disease: In this groundbreaking approach, the process begins with extracting neuronal stem cells directly from the patient.

These cells, possessing the remarkable potential to develop into various types of nerve cells, are then cultivated and nurtured within the controlled environment of a laboratory setting.

Here, under carefully monitored conditions, they are coaxed to multiply and differentiate into the specific neuronal cells crucially needed to combat the effects of Parkinson's.

This intricate cultivation process ensures the growth of healthy, functional neurons tailored to the individual's unique biological makeup.

Once deemed mature and ready for action, these revitalized neurons are delicately re-implanted back into the patient's body, precisely targeting the affected regions of the brain.

Through this innovative therapy, the aim is not only to alleviate the symptoms of Parkinson's Disease but also to potentially halt its progression.

By replenishing the brain with rejuvenated neurons, stem cell therapy holds the promise of restoring lost function, improving motor skills, and enhancing the overall quality of life for those grappling with this debilitating condition.

As research in stem cell therapy continues to advance, the possibilities for its application in treating a myriad of neurological disorders, including Parkinson's Disease, offer a glimmer of hope on the horizon of medical science.

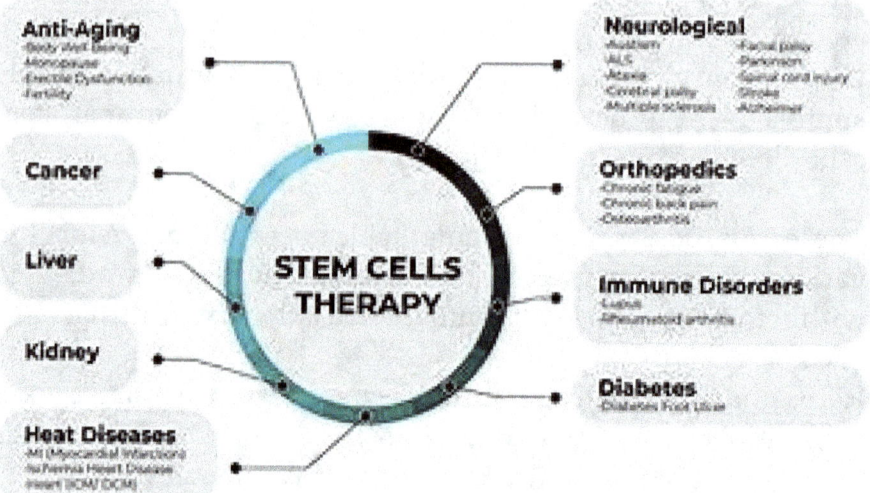

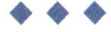

Embarking on a Stem-tastic Adventure: The Magical Journey of Stem Cell Therapy!

Picture this: In the land of Ouchies and Boo Boos, there's a special potion that turns frowns upside down.

Let's zoom into the story of Timmy, a brave young knight battling the mighty dragon called Parkinson's Disease!

First off, Timmy's doctors whisk him away to the lab, where they perform some super sneaky moves to pluck out his magical cells, called neuronal stem cells.

These cells are like little wizards that can grow into all sorts of cool nerve cells.

Now, hold onto your hats, because here comes the fun part: these magical cells get sent to the lab's wizardry department, where they're given VIP treatment.

They're fed the yummiest nutrients and put under a special spell to multiply and transform into exactly the kind of cells Timmy's brain needs to defeat the dragon.

Once these super-powered cells are all grown up and ready for action, it's time for the grand finale! Timmy's doctors take these freshly brewed neurons and gently tuck them back into his brain, like planting seeds in a garden.

And guess what?

With these new wizard cells on the scene, Timmy's brain gets its mojo back! Suddenly, moving and grooving becomes a breeze, and Timmy can go back to slaying imaginary dragons with his trusty sword.

So, youngsters, remember when it feels like the dragons of sickness are breathing down your neck, there's always a magical potion waiting to turn the tables and make you the hero of your own story!

Semaglutide: For Diabetic and Weight Control.

Get ready to chuckle with Semaglutide, the Whiz-Bang Wonder Drug of Diabetes Delights!

Imagine a medicine so cool, it's like having a secret agent battling diabetes right inside your body! Meet Semaglutide, aka Ozempic and Rybelsus, with a half-life so long, that it's practically on vacation for a week!

Now, let's talk about dosing - it's like following a recipe for a magic potion. You start with a teensy-weensy dose of 0.25 mg once a week, just to test the waters.

If your tummy doesn't throw a tantrum, you can level up to 0.5 mg. And if your body's feeling like a champ, why not go for the gold with 1 mg a week?

But wait, there's more! Semaglutide isn't just about keeping sugar levels in check - it's also a secret weapon against pesky pounds. That's right, folks, it's like having a personal trainer for your metabolism!

Now, onto the comedy of side effects! Nausea, vomiting, and diarrhea - it's like your body's throwing a wild party, but you're not invited! And the more Semaglutide you take, the more it cranks up the wackiness!

But hold onto your hats, folks - there's a catch! If your family tree has a whiff of Medullary Thyroid Carcinoma or the tongue-twisting Multiple Endocrine Neoplasia Syndrome Type

2, Semaglutide like, "Sorry, pal, you're not on the guest list!"

But hey, despite the bellyaches and the family drama, people are lining up to get their hands on Semaglutide. Doctors are even prescribing it for folks who just want to shed a few extra pounds - it's like having a weight-loss coach on the speed dial!

Just one little snag - if you're not in the diabetes club, using Semaglutide for weight loss is like crashing a party without an invite. Sure, it's legal, but your wallet might take a hit bigger than a sumo wrestler!

So, unless you're ready to splurge $11,000 a month, you might want to stick to an old-fashioned diet and exercise... or invest in some bigger pants!

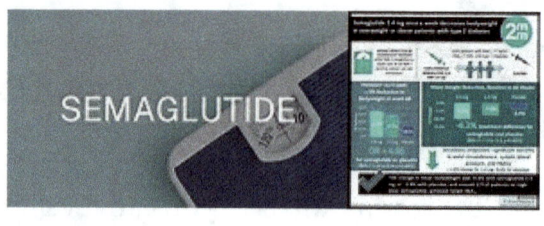

◆ ◆ ◆

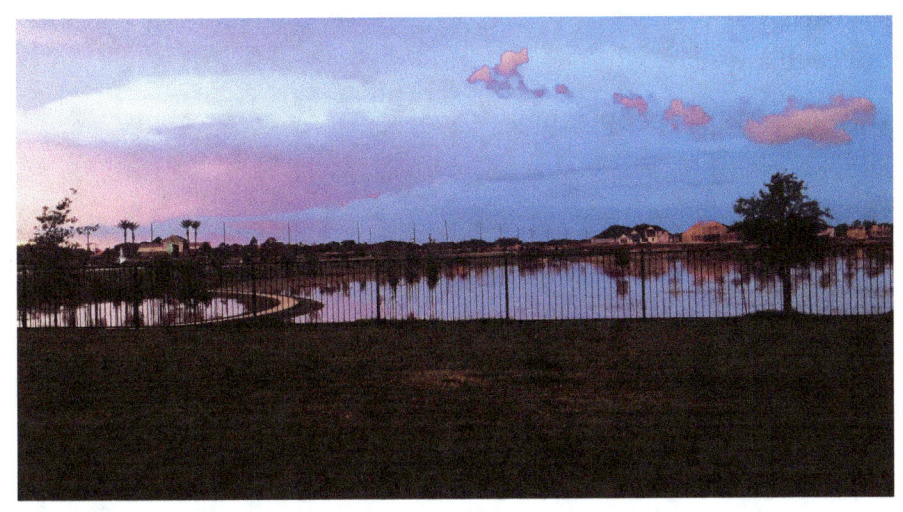

CHAPTER 11

GOD's Love Anyway

A positive belief system for Eternal Life
GOD's love- A beacon of hope for Eternal Life

ANYWAY

People are often
 unreasonable, illogical, and self-centered.

Forgive them anyway.

If you are kind, people may
accuse you of selfish ulterior motives,

Be kind anyway.

If you are successful, you
will win some false friends and some true enemies.

Succeed anyway.

If you are frank, people may
cheat you.

Be honest anyway,

What you spend years
building, someone could destroy overnight.

Build anyway!

If you find serenity and
happiness, they may be jealous.

Be happy anyway.

The good you do today,
people will often forget tomorrow.

Do good anyway.

Give the world the best you
have, and it may never be enough!

Give the best you have gotten anyway.

You see, in the final
analysis, it's between you and God,

it is never between you and them anyway,

Remember, it is never merely about them, but about your connection with the Divine, anyhow.

LIVE LONGER LOVE LONGER PART 3

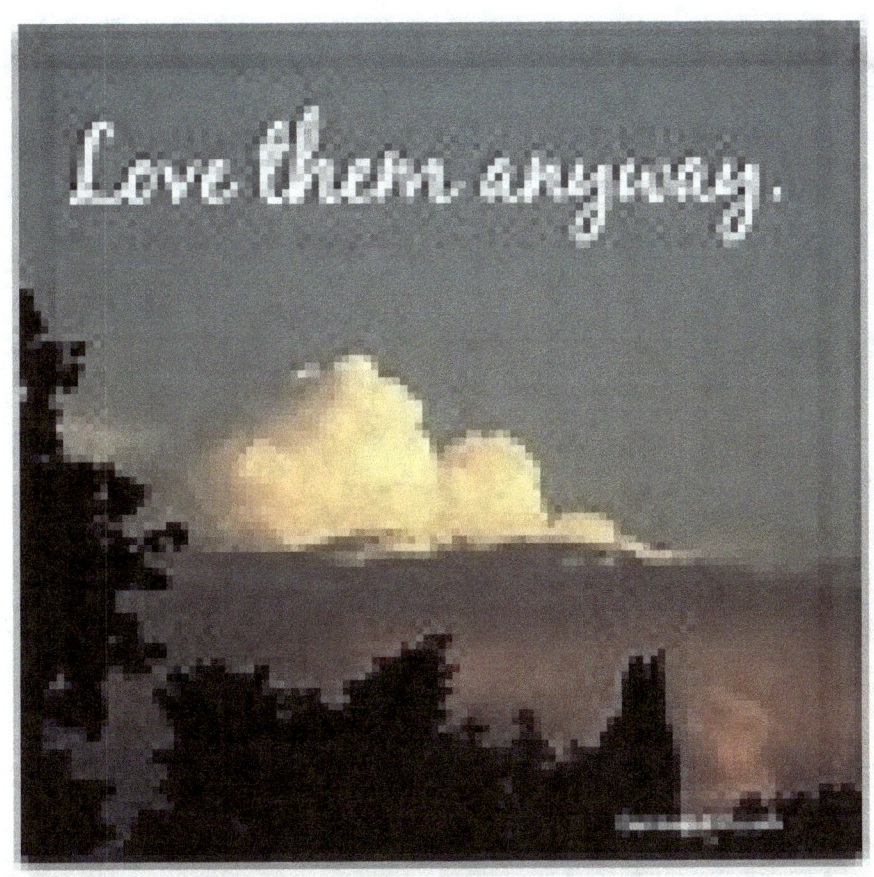

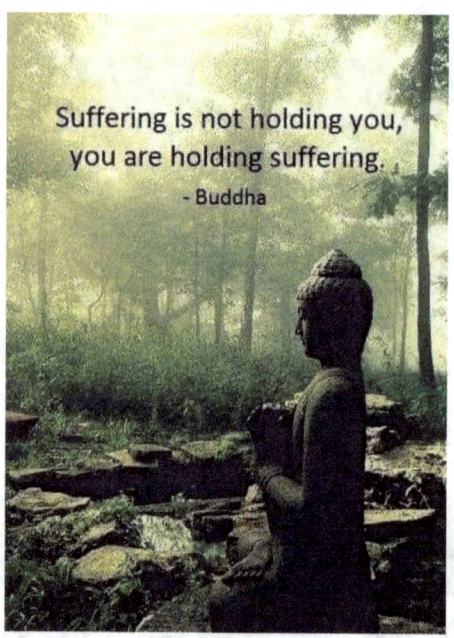

Spiritual Weaponry: Combating Deception

In his insightful work, "Defeating Deception: A Spiritual Approach to Life and Health," Dr. Gayden emphasizes the significance of spirituality in combating the adversities of life, including aging.

He presents an empowering perspective, viewing age as a treatable condition rather than an inevitable decline.

Central to Dr. Gaydon's approach is the "Five Weapons Against Satan," tools aimed at warding off deception and negativity in our lives. At the forefront is the power of the Word of God, a potent weapon against temptation and falsehood.

Drawing inspiration from biblical passages, He highlights the efficacy of vocalizing scripture to fortify one's spirit against the trials of life.

Referencing the teachings of Jesus Christ, He underscores the transformative power of proclaiming, "It is written," in moments of temptation.

Through verses such as John 8:36 and Ephesians 6:17, he illustrates the sword-like potency of the Word of God in dispelling darkness and guiding believers toward freedom and clarity.

Moreover, He delves into the dynamic nature of the Word, as depicted in Hebrews 4:12 and John 1:14, emphasizing its ability to penetrate the depths of the human soul and effect profound change.

He illustrates how the Word, likened to seeds in the parable of the Sower (Luke 8:4-15), has the potential to yield abundant growth when sown in receptive hearts.

In confronting the father of lies, as Jesus referred to the devil (John 8:44), He stresses the importance of arming oneself with knowledge, as elucidated in Hosea 4:6.

He asserts that ignorance paves the path to destruction, whereas the enlightenment found in the Word of God serves as a shield against deception's allure.

Ultimately, "Defeating Deception" serves as a beacon of hope, guiding readers toward a deeper spiritual understanding and empowering them to confront life's challenges with faith and resilience.
Dr. Gaydon's insights offer not only a path to spiritual

enlightenment but also a roadmap to enhanced well-being and longevity.

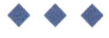

Harnessing the Power of Praise: A Path to Physical and Emotional Healing.

In his illuminating discourse, Dr. John Gaydon Jr. MD unveils the transformative potential of praise as a formidable weapon against afflictions like tumors and depression, fostering holistic well-being.

With reverence, He elucidates the unique potency of praise, offering it as a sacred offering to God.

Drawing from Isaiah 42:10-13, He illustrates the majestic response of the divine to heartfelt praises. He reveals how God, akin to a mighty warrior, is stirred to action when His children raise their voices in joyful adulation, triumphing over adversities with a resounding victory.

Through the biblical account in 2 Chronicles 20:1-22, He exemplifies the miraculous intervention spurred by praise. When faced with overwhelming odds, King Jehoshaphat dispatched singers to herald God's praises. Their worship catalyzed divine intervention, leading to the supernatural deliverance of the besieged nation.

Likewise, in Acts 16:16-40, He recounts the awe-inspiring narrative of Paul and Silas. Amidst persecution and imprisonment, their steadfast devotion manifested in hymns of praise.

Miraculously, their praises precipitated the miraculous liberation of not only themselves but also their fellow prisoners, underscoring the profound impact of worship in adversity.

In weaving together these biblical anecdotes, He emphasizes the intrinsic link between praise and spiritual fortitude.

Quoting Isaiah 61:3 and Nehemiah 8:10, he portrays praise as a transformative garment, replacing despair with radiant joy and endowing believers with divine strength.

"Harnessing the Power of Praise" serves as a clarion call to believers, inviting them to embrace the transcendent efficacy of praise in navigating life's trials.

Through heartfelt adoration, He asserts, individuals can unlock the boundless reservoirs of God's grace, finding solace, healing, and empowerment in communion with the Divine.

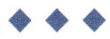

Unleashing the Authority of Jesus Christ for Healing

In his illuminating discourse on the authority of Jesus Christ, Dr. Gaydon unveils a miraculous weapon for restoring physical health: the authoritative command in the name of Jesus Christ.

With unwavering faith, He elucidates the profound efficacy of prayer coupled with the commanding power bestowed by Christ.

Citing the words of Jesus from Mark 16:17-18, He underscores the promise of healing for those who believe, empowering believers to lay hands on the sick and command restoration in Jesus' name.

He emphasizes that Christ, as affirmed in Matthew 28:18, possesses ultimate authority over all realms, including sickness and infirmity.

Moreover, drawing from Luke 10:19, He elucidates the transference of this authority to believers, granting them power over the enemy's dominion.

Through examples such as Jesus' rebuke of the fever in Peter's mother-in-law (Luke 4) and His calming of the storm (Luke 8), He illustrates the transformative potential of speaking with authority in alignment with Christ's teachings.

Reflecting on the creative power of spoken word, Dr. Gaydon references the biblical account of God speaking the world into existence in Genesis 1, underscoring the inherent potency of verbal command in shaping reality.

Furthermore, he highlights the efficacy of fervent prayer, as emphasized in Hebrews 5:7 and James 5:16, stressing the importance of earnest supplication and bold declarations in accessing divine intervention.

In reassurance, He invokes scriptures such as Luke 10:19, 2 Timothy 1:7, and 1 John 4:4, affirming believers' inheritance of power, love, and soundness of mind in Christ.

He encourages readers to embrace their divine authority and confront challenges with confidence, knowing that the indwelling presence of Christ within them surpasses any opposing force in the world.

"Unleashing the Authority of Jesus Christ for Healing" stands as a testament to the transformative potential of faith-filled prayer and authoritative proclamation, offering hope and empowerment to those seeking restoration and wholeness in body and spirit.

The Dynamic Force of Prayer

In his insightful exploration, Dr. John Gaydon Jr. MD underscores the transformative potency of fervent prayer, highlighting its inherent energy and efficacy, even when uttered aloud.

He advocates for the holistic application of all five spiritual weapons against the wiles of Satan to navigate life's myriad challenges successfully.

Drawing from 1 Thessalonians 5:17, He emphasizes the directive to maintain a continual posture of prayer, harnessing its enduring power in all facets of life.

Moreover, referencing Philippians 4:6, He exhorts believers to exchange anxiety for fervent supplication, entrusting every concern into the hands of God through prayer.

He underscores the transformative potential of prayer as a conduit for receiving the living water of the Holy Spirit, as depicted in John 7:37-39.

In synthesizing these biblical admonitions, He underscores the holistic impact of fervent prayer on spiritual well-being, urging believers to engage in constant communion with the Divine.

Through fervent prayer, he contends, individuals can unlock reservoirs of divine grace, finding solace, guidance, and empowerment in the presence of God.

"The Dynamic Force of Prayer" serves as a beacon of hope, guiding believers towards a deeper spiritual communion and empowering them to navigate life's challenges with faith and resilience.

Dr. Gaydon's insights offer not only a path to spiritual enlightenment but also a roadmap to enhanced spiritual vitality and communion with the Divine.

Fortifying Faith: A Spiritual Arsenal for Life's Challenges

In his insightful discourse on the potency of faith, Dr. John Gaydon Jr. MD unveils the shield of faith as a formidable weapon against life's adversities.

Drawing from biblical wisdom, He underscores the pivotal role of faith in navigating the complexities of existence and fortifying one's spiritual resilience.

Citing Romans 10:17, He elucidates the foundational principle that faith is cultivated through exposure to the Word of God, underscoring the transformative power of scriptural engagement in strengthening one's spiritual convictions.

Referencing Jesus' teaching in Luke 17, He highlights the exponential potential of even the smallest seed of faith, urging believers to trust in God's unfathomable ability to bring about miraculous outcomes.

Echoing the exhortation in Ephesians 6, He emphasizes the imperative to wield the shield of faith as a defense against the attacks of the enemy, safeguarding one's spiritual integrity and well-being.

Moreover, drawing from James 1:6-7, He underscores the necessity of unwavering faith in prayer, cautioning against the destabilizing effects of doubt and wavering conviction.

In addressing life's multifaceted challenges, He advocates for a holistic approach, employing all five spiritual weapons to combat the onslaught of adversity and secure life extension and quality.

For relational challenges, He advocates intentional forgiveness as a transformative act, releasing the burden of resentment and fostering spiritual liberation.

In moments of spiritual turmoil, He encourages believers to shift their focus from problems to God, anchoring themselves in the unshakable certainty of divine providence.

For physical ailments, Dr. Gaydon invokes the healing authority of Jesus Christ, leveraging the power of scripture and prayer to invite miraculous interventions.

In addressing emotional distress, He echoes the call to redirect attention toward God's steadfast presence, finding solace and strength in divine communion.

Finally, for financial concerns, He invokes the promise of divine provision as articulated in Philippians 4:19, encouraging believers to trust in God's abundant provision.

"Fortifying Faith" serves as a guiding beacon for believers, equipping them with spiritual wisdom and practical strategies to overcome life's trials and emerge victorious in their faith journey.

Through unwavering trust in God and diligent application of spiritual principles, believers can navigate life's challenges with resilience, confidence, and unwavering faith.

Daily Mindful Meditation for Wellness

Daily Spiritual Reflection

(1) Embrace a mindset of positivity through mindful awareness to enhance your immune system.

(2) Cultivate bodily relaxation and mental tranquility.

(3) An offering towards elevating consciousness to a higher realm.

Daily Edgar Cayce Meditation Adventure for Youngsters!

(A) Energize Your Body: Imagine yourself becoming stronger and healthier every day.

(B) Brighten Your Mind: Picture your thoughts shining like stars in the sky.

(C) Explore Your Spirit: Close your eyes and feel the magic inside you.

(1) Build Your Shield: Pretend you're a superhero putting on your invisible shield to keep distractions away. Say, "I am protected by love and goodness."

(2) Find Inner Peace: Imagine your worries floating away like bubbles. Keep practicing until you feel light and free inside.

(3) Let Your Spirit Soar: Trust your inner superhero to guide you. Your dreams and feelings are like secret messages from a wise friend.

(4) Connect with the Universe: Imagine you're talking to the stars and they're whispering back to you. Feel the love and peace surrounding you.

Remember, using your imagination and staying motivated helps you talk to the universe. Just like a friend knocking on your door, open your heart to the magic of meditation.

And don't forget, taking quiet time each day is like pressing pause on the busy world, giving you a chance to connect with the amazing energy all around you.

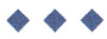

The Kingdom of Heaven

Let's Explore the Kingdom of Heaven!

Did you know that the kingdom of heaven is right inside us? It's like having a magical place in our hearts that grows bigger and brighter when we're kind and helpful to others.

Imagine feeling the joy of heaven when you do good things and make the world a better place. It's like having a special awareness of the love and goodness around us.

When we think good thoughts and use kind words, it's like planting seeds of love that grow into beautiful deeds. We can fill our minds with thoughts of love, mercy, gentleness, and forgiveness, just like Jesus taught us.

The key is to connect with the universal consciousness, where we feel one with God and all living things. It's like tuning into a special radio station where we can hear messages of hope and wisdom.

Sometimes, if we listen closely to our hearts, we might even see things beyond what our eyes can see or hear things beyond what our ears can hear. It's like having superpowers of seeing, hearing, and feeling with our souls.

But we have to be careful! Negative thoughts and selfishness can block our connection to heaven. Instead, we should spread love and kindness wherever we go, without expecting anything in return.

So, let's open our hearts to the light of Christ and shine brightly with love, patience, understanding, and forgiveness. That's how we bring a little piece of heaven right here on Earth!

◆ ◆ ◆

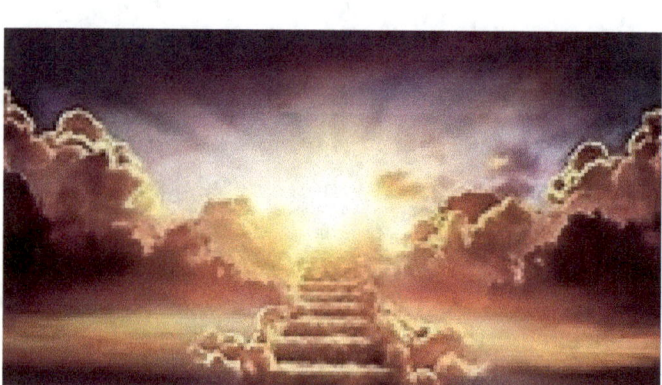

Prayer is Talking to GOD.

Prayer: a chat with GOD

Prayer is like having a chat with God, where we share our

thoughts, hopes, and worries with Him.

Meditation: Listening to God

Meditation is like tuning into God's voice, where we quiet our minds and listen to the gentle whispers deep within us.

Dreams: God's Messages

Sometimes, God speaks to us through dreams. We should pay attention to the messages and meanings hidden within them.

Powerful suggestions: Lifting our Spirits.

We can use powerful words to lift our spirits and connect with the universal mind and spirit of God.

Being Still: Allowing God's Will

When we feel the presence of God's spirit, we can surrender our desires and say, "Not my will, but yours." Then, we simply let go and allow God's will to guide us.

At-Onement with God: Our Purpose

Being at one with God means being companions with the Creator, which is the true purpose of our lives.

The Sin of Self-gratification

The biggest mistake we can make is being selfish and only seeking to satisfy our desires. Instead, we should strive to live in harmony with God's will and serve others with love and compassion.

Edgar Cayce's Meditation Method

Preparation Steps

Before starting, ensure that your purpose in life aligns with serving the greater good, following the example of Jesus Christ.

Head and Neck Exercises

Begin by gently moving your head and neck to release tension. Tilt your head forward, backward, and side to side three times each.

Protective Prayer

As you approach the divine presence, surround yourself with the protective love of God-consciousness and Christ-consciousness. Feel the power of this protection as you recite the Lord's Prayer.

Breathing Techniques

Practice deep breathing to calm your mind and body. Inhale deeply through one nostril and exhale through the mouth, then switch nostrils. Repeat seven cycles of normal breathing.

The Rising Incantation

Chant the syllables "Ah, A, E, I, O, U, M" with your head drawn back, activating the autonomic nervous system to bring balance and fulfillment to your life.

Physical Preparation

Find a comfortable place, ideally at 2 am, and perform stretching exercises to awaken your body's energy.

Breathing Exercises

Lie down with your hands on your stomach and focus on removing any earthly distractions. Surrender control to your autonomic nervous system.

Surrender to God's Will

Draw your head back as you sense the presence of God, affirming, "Not my will, but yours be done in and through me."

Silent Abiding

Enter a state of silence, balancing the energies throughout your body and mind.

Transitioning From Meditation

As you conclude, maintain the mindset of embodying Jesus's thoughts, words, and actions for the next 24 hours. Edgar Cayce's Method of Meditation.

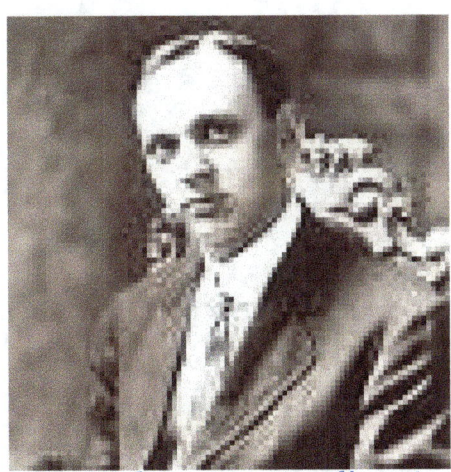

https://edgarcayce.org/edgar-cayce/readings/meditation-prayer/

◆ ◆ ◆

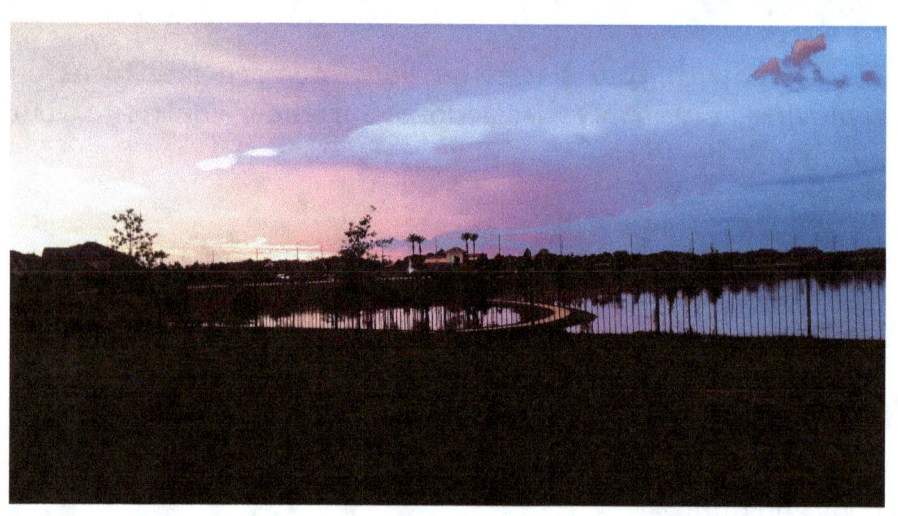

CHAPTER 12

Diet for Higher Consciousness'

Elevate Your Consciousness with This Dietary Plan

Morning Boost
(1) Kick-start your day with a refreshing glass of citrus juice:
(a) Blend orange juice with a hint of lemon or lime.
(b) Indulge in the tangy goodness of grapefruit juice.

(2) Enjoy the creamy yolk of a softly boiled egg (chilled for extra delight).

(3) Savor toasted rye bread.

(4) Accompany your breakfast with a cup of invigorating coffee or tea.

Rotate Every 24 Hours:

(1) Delight in well-cooked steel-cut oats.

(2) Embrace a warm bowl of cereal with a dash of butter and salt.

(3) Sweeten if necessary with honey or brown sugar.

Midday Feast

(1) Relish a colorful array of fresh raw vegetables drizzled with red wine vinegar and oil.

(2) Opts for vegetables grown above ground for optimal nutrition:
- Asparagus, broccoli, green beans, spinach, mushrooms, cabbage, cauliflower, Brussels sprouts, eggplant, celery, and leafy greens.

(3) Minimize intake of starchy vegetables such as corn, beans, lima beans, peas, potatoes, sweet potatoes, and winter squash.

(4) Warm up with a comforting vegetable soup or broth (avoiding pork, fried meats, and red meat).

(5) Pair your meal with fish, poultry, or lamb alongside a side of fresh raw vegetables.

Evening Fare

(1) Enjoy cooked vegetables seasoned with vinegar.

(2) Indulge in your choice of fish, poultry, or lamb.

(3) Satisfy your sweet tooth with plain Knox gelatin infused with juice or vegetables to retain vital nutrients from your meal.

After breakfast, keep yourself busy with work. After lunch, take a well-deserved rest, Before dinner, unwind with a glass of red wine and a slice of black bread, and post-dinner, enjoy a leisurely stroll for a mile.

Gift For the Day: Happy Life Tips

Here's a fun list of things to do to keep you feeling awesome and happy every day!

1. Be like a graceful dancer, moving through life with style and charm!

2. Learn about how your brain and body work together like superheroes! Imagine your immune system as an army fighting off bad guys!

3. Believe in good things like magic and kindness. It's like having a superpower!

4. Live every day like it's a big adventure waiting to happen!

5. Pay attention to the different seasons, like a nature detective!

6. Get a little sunshine every day to recharge your happy

batteries!

7. Try to have dreams where you can fly and do all sorts of cool stuff!

8. Look for beauty everywhere, like in a colorful sunset or a cute puppy!

9. Remember, it's not the things that make you happy, it's the people and experiences that matter most!

10. Don't worry about what others think about you, just be yourself! But if someone gives you good advice, listen!

11. Keep your brain muscles strong by learning new things every day!

12. Challenge yourself to try new things, like learning to juggle or riding a unicycle!

13. Always look on the bright side of life, like a happy little sunbeam!

14. Say thank you for all the good things in your life, big and small!

15. Share your toys, your snacks, and your smile with someone who needs it!

16. Be honest and true, like a brave knight or a wise wizard!

17. Take care of yourself by eating healthy foods and getting plenty of sleep and exercise!

18. Write down your thoughts and feelings in a special journal, like a secret treasure map of your heart!

19. Don't ever stop doing things you love, even when you grow up!

20. Keep your mind open to new ideas and adventures, like a door that's always ready to swing open!

21. Remember the 4 Cs: Challenge yourself, Commit to your goals, Stay Curious, and Let your creativity shine!

22. If you have a partner, remember to be fair, give them space, and have fun together!

23. Laughing is like giving your heart a big warm hug! So smile, because it's good for you!

24. Don't get stuck doing boring stuff all the time! Go out and play tennis, ride horses, or even try surfing!

25. Doing nice things for others is like giving your heart a big high-five!

26. Use happy words and spread joy wherever you go, like a happy superhero!

27. If work stresses you out, take breaks, listen to music, and imagine yourself as a superhero fighting stress monsters!

28. Make lists of all the cool things you want to do, like climbing mountains or learning to bake cookies!

29. Learn how to save lives with CPR, just like a superhero!

30. Having youngsters is like having your little team of superheroes to play with and love!

31. Pets are like furry best friends who make life more fun and full of love! Plus, they make you go for walks and keep you company when you're feeling lonely!

Personal Hygiene: Hygiene Essential for Senior

Maintain Your Grown-Up Glow! Forget the days of just grabbing any old soap and calling it a day. It's time for some serious adulting when it comes to personal hygiene!

Here's your essential toolkit for keeping yourself fresh and fabulous:

1. Tired of sensitivity? Check out whiteningpowerswabs.com for tooth whitening that won't make you wince.

2. Brighten up your smile with the latest Colgate Optic White Toothpaste.

3. For on-the-go whitening, try Crest Whitening Emulsions.

4. Scrub-a-dub-dub with Nivea Body Wash or get that extra kick with Axe Body Wash.

5. Give your locs some love with Garnier Fructis Treat Plumping Conditioner.

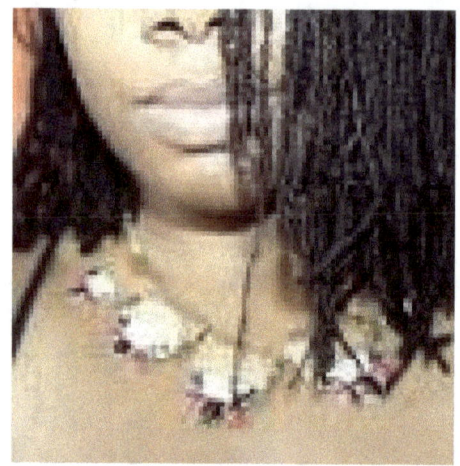

6. Stay fresh with aluminum-free deodorant infused with essential oils.

7. Keep those wrinkles at bay with L'Oreal Paris Revitalift Triple Power Retinol Serum.

8. Say goodbye to dry skin with LZRr 3% Pure Retinol Night Cream.

9. Say hello to a flake-free scalp with Head & Shoulders Clinical Strength Dandruff Defense Shampoo (or try out that fancy pine nut oil option).

10. Protect your skin from the Aussie sun with Blue Lizard Australian Sunscreen.

11. And don't forget about your eyes! Treat them right with Thera Tears Dry Eye Therapy.

Because being a grown-up means taking care of yourself, from head to toe!

◆ ◆ ◆

COVID Rules

In the Ongoing Battle Against COVID: The Rules of Survival

As the world teeters on the edge of uncertainty, one thing remains clear: survival depends on our wits and adherence to the rules.

Here's your guide to navigating the treacherous terrain of pandemic living:

1. Stay vigilant, stay protected. Keep your vaccinations up to date, for they are the armor shielding you from the invisible enemy.

2. Don your mask like a warrior dons their helm. Seek out only the highest quality, CDC-certified N-95 masks—their efficacy may mean the difference between triumph and defeat.

3. In the face of uncertainty, arm yourself with knowledge. Rapid antigen tests serve as your trusty sword, aiding in swift diagnosis when the enemy strikes.

4. Beware the shadows that lurk within. Improve indoor ventilation to ward off the encroaching threat, for stagnant air breeds danger.

5. Prepare your arsenal with care. Keep antiviral pills close at hand, bestowed upon you by the guardians of health—the local health department. They may serve as your last line of defense in the heat of battle.

6. Should fate cast its shadow upon you and the test reveal the enemy's presence, fear not. Heed the call of the CDC, and follow

their latest guidelines as a map through the darkness, guiding you safely through the storm.

In this ever-shifting landscape, only those who remain vigilant, adaptable, and steadfast in their resolve shall emerge victorious.

Let us stand together, united in our fight against the unseen foe.

Safety/Peace Of Mind

Keep Calm and Secure On!
Alrighty, folks, let's talk about safety and peace of mind because adulting isn't just about paying bills and pretending to know what you're doing.

First up, home security and medical alerts. Check out lifelock360norton.com for some serious peace of mind. Think of it as your digital bouncer keeping out the riff-raff.

Now, emergencies happen, whether it's a zombie apocalypse or just a really bad hair day.

So, let's get you sorted with a mobile supply kit. Think snacks, water, a flashlight, and maybe some emergency cash for when the vending machine eats your last dollar.

Next on the agenda: end-of-life decisions.

Yeah, it's morbid, but hey, it's better to be prepared than caught with your pants down. Get yourself a will, a power of attorney (because who doesn't want someone else to make decisions for them?), and a living will answer the big questions like "Do you want to be zapped back to life or left to chill?"

Oh, and don't forget about your medical info.

Stick it on your computer and upload it to the cloud. And just in case your computer decides to join the circus and run away, scan those docs onto a USB keychain. Because you never know when you'll need to prove that you're not a robot.

Stay safe, stay sane, and remember, it's all fun and games until someone forgets to back up their medical history!

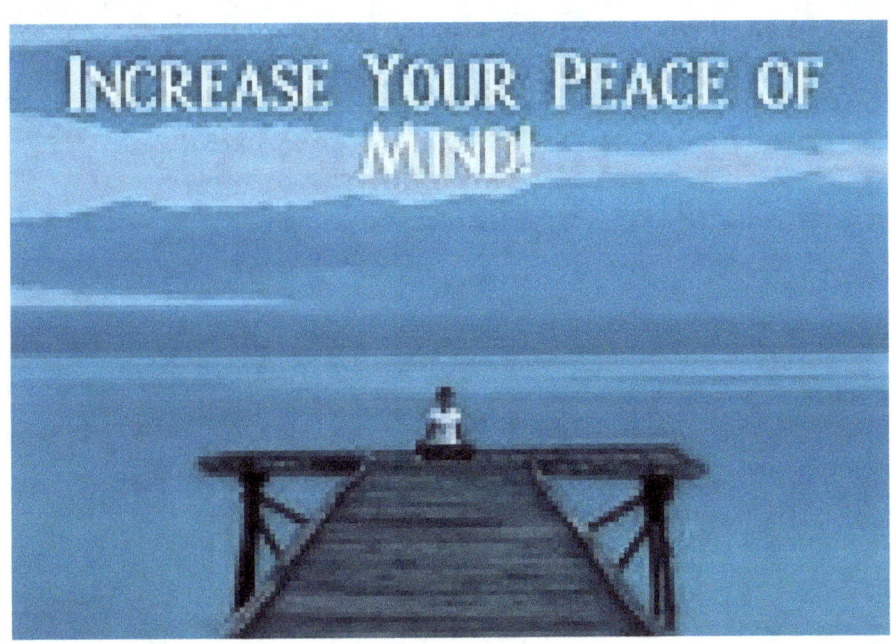

References and Glossary

Ah, behold the treasure trove of wisdom and silliness known as the "References and Glossary" from the first installment of our series, "Live Longer Love Longer: Age is a Treatable Disease."

Get ready to dive into a world where science meets satire, where references are as entertaining as they are informative!

General References:
1. Anderson, R. N. (2000). The Ten Leading Causes of Death in the U.S.: Final Data for 2000.
To
63. Ames, B. N., Elson-Schwab, I., & Silver, E. A. (2002). High-Dose Vitamin Therapy Stimulates Variant Enzymes with Decreased Coenzyme Binding Affinity: Relevance to Genetic Diseases and Polymorphisms. The American Journal of Nutrition, Apr; 75(4), 616-658.

Glossary: Word List: Tricky Book Terms.

Book series of "Live Longer Love Longer" by this author:

Book Title: Age is a treatable disease Kindle Edition
Amazon store Link:
https://www.amazon.com/dp/B0CY69VBTR

Book Title: "Live Longer Love Longer Part 2"
Amazon store Link:

HTTPs://www.amazon.com/dp/B0CYJCRXXL

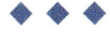

EPILOGUE

Hilarious Guide to Eternal Youth

Title: Live Longer Love Longer Part 3: Age is a Treatable Disease - A Hilariously Insightful Journey to Eternal Youth

If you're like me and dread the idea of aging like a soggy banana, then "Live Longer Love Longer Part 3: Age is a Treatable Disease" is your ultimate salvation wrapped in a hilarious package!

Dr. Quirky takes you on a rollercoaster ride through the science of staying young, all while keeping you in stitches with his witty commentary.

From the absurdity of considering aging a medical condition to the wild world of gene technologies, this book leaves no anti-aging stone unturned.

But what truly sets this book apart is its ability to balance scientific insight with side-splitting humor. Who knew that discussing stem cells and regenerative medicine could be so entertaining?

Dr. Quirky's knack for turning complex concepts into digestible nuggets of comedic gold is nothing short of genius.

Not only does "Age is a Treatable Disease" provide a roadmap to defying Father Time, but it also delivers a hefty dose of optimism about the future of aging.

Who wouldn't want to live in a world where getting older means getting healthier and happier?

And let's not forget the practical advice sprinkled throughout, from dietary tips for higher consciousness to the importance of daily meditation.

Dr. Quirky's holistic approach to longevity ensures that readers not only extend their years but also their quality of life.

So, if you're ready to laugh, learn, and maybe even shed a tear of joy at the thought of a future without wrinkles, do yourself a favor and dive into this book.

Your future self will thank you for it, preferably with a youthful glow and a hearty chuckle.

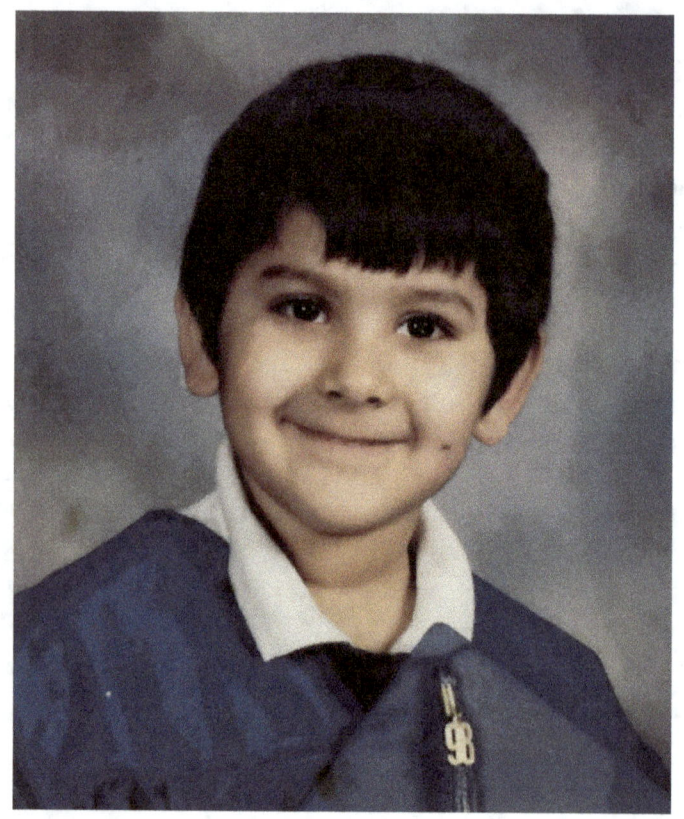

Umar Syed RIP 1992-2016

Umar Syed Foundation Corporation is a dynamic private foundation based in Baytown, TX, dedicated to championing education, healthcare, and scientific advancement for underserved children in our community.

For inquiries, reach out to us via email at Medicaltower@gmail.com or send mail to our office address: 5714 Comal Park Ct, Houston, Texas 77059

Together, let's build a brighter future through education, health, and science for all.

Warm regards,

[Umar Syed Foundation Team]

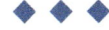